ACKNOWLEDGMENTS

Writing this book has reminded me to be grateful for the many gifts I have received from others.

I would like to acknowledge my parents, Milton and Frances Williams, who taught me to have faith and to persevere.

My mentors and teachers have also inspired me, especially Alyce Foley, an unforgettable teacher and counselor who had a strong influence on my decision to become a psychiatric nurse. Hildegard Peplau, a woman of incredible strength and dignity, taught me that every interaction with a client is an opportunity for growth and that effective communication is always challenging and interesting.

My students have prompted me to write this book each time they challenged me to explain myself and to answer the question "What is therapeutic interaction?" I hope the explanations and examples in this book help to clarify the nuances of this sometimes elusive but critical component of nursing practice.

Christine L. Williams, DNSc, RN, BC

I would like to acknowledge my mother, Marjorie Hagen Davis, who was the first nurse in my life, and my twin sister, Susan Doughty, RN, MS, NP, CS, who I believe to be a consummate role model for all nurses. Her skills as a women's health nurse practitioner and critical care clinical specialist are emulated by all who come in contact with her.

Carol M. Davis, PT, EdD, MS, FAPTA

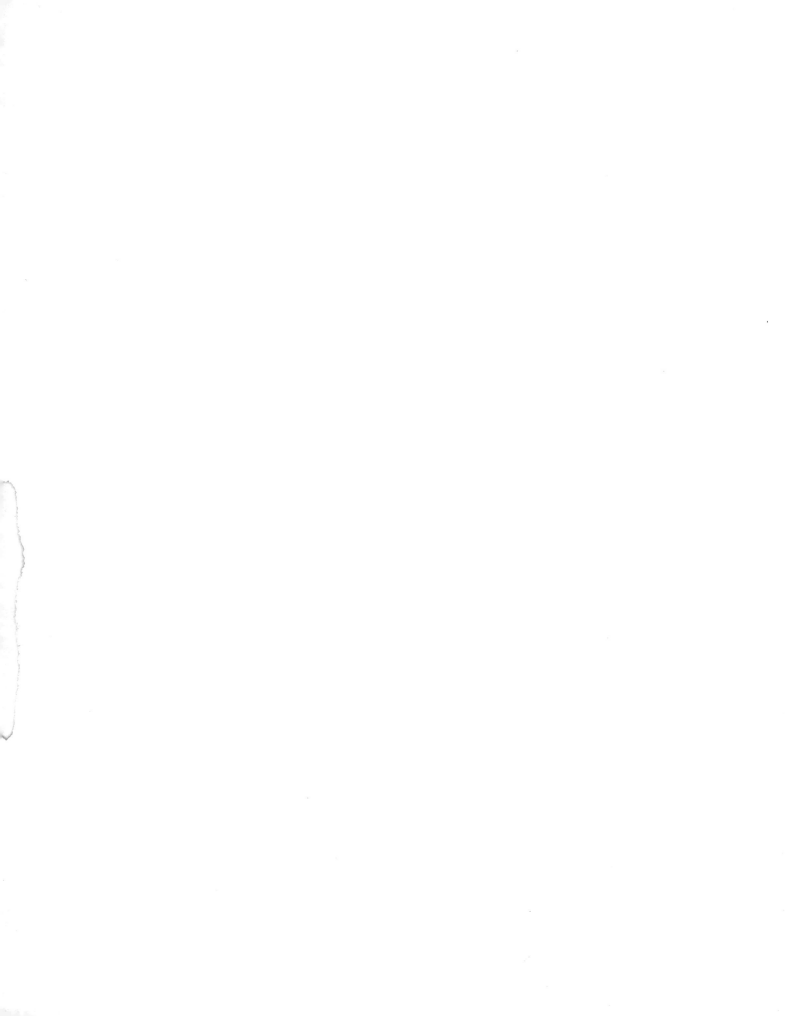

CONTENTS

Instructors: *Therapeutic Interaction in Nursing* Instructor's Manual is also available from Jones and Bartlett Publishers. To obtain the Instructor's Manual, please visit this text's catalog page at *http://www.jbpub.com.*

Therapeutic Interaction in Nursing

Christine L. Williams, DNSc, RN, BC
Associate Professor
University of Miami
School of Nursing
Coral Gables, Fla

with

Carol M. Davis, PT, EdD, MS, FAPTA
Department of Physical Therapy
University of Miami
School of Medicine
Coral Gables, Fla

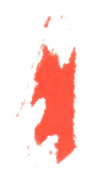

JONES AND BARTLETT PUBLISHERS
Sudbury, Massachusetts
BOSTON   TORONTO   LONDON   SINGAPORE

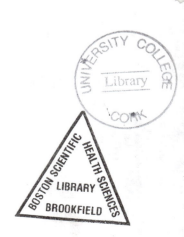

World Headquarters
Jones and Bartlett Publishers
40 Tall Pine Drive
Sudbury, MA 01776
978-443-5000
info@jbpub.com
www.jbpub.com

Jones and Bartlett Publishers Canada
2406 Nikanna Road
Mississauga, ON L5C 2W6
CANADA

Jones and Bartlett Publishers International
Barb House, Barb Mews
London W6 7PA
UK

Jones and Bartlett's books and products are available through most bookstores and online booksellers. To contact Jones and Bartlett Publishers directly, call 800-832-0034, fax 978-443-8000, or visit ourwebsite www.jbpub.com.

Substantial discounts on bulk quantities of Jones and Bartlett's publications are available to corporations, professional associations, and other qualified organizations. For details and specific discount information, contact the special sales department at Jones and Bartlett via the above contact information or send an email to specialsales@jbpub.com.

ISBN 0-7637-3744-5

Production Credits
Acquisitions Editor: Kevin Sullivan
Production Director: Amy Rose
Associate Editor: Amy Sibley
Production Assistant: Kate Hennessy
Marketing Manager: Emily Ekle
Production Specialist: Colleen Halloran
Manufacturing and Inventory Coordinator: Amy Bacus
Printing and Binding: Courier Stoughton

Printed in the United States of America
09 08 07 06 05   10 9 8 7 6 5 4 3 2 1

DEDICATION

To my beloved daughter, Lauren.

ABOUT THE AUTHORS

Christine L. Williams, DNSc, RN, BC, graduated from Fitchburg State College in 1971 with an undergraduate degree in nursing. She completed a master's degree in Advanced Psychiatric Nursing at Rutgers University in 1973 and received a Doctor of Nursing Science degree from Boston University in 1986. She worked as a staff nurse in psychiatric nursing and later as a Clinical Specialist in Psychiatric Nursing before beginning a career as an educator and researcher. In 1994 she was appointed associate professor at the School of Nursing, University of Miami. Currently, she specializes in psychiatric mental health nursing and gerontological nursing and she has combined academic teaching and clinical supervision of students with an outstanding research record. She has presented many papers to national and international audiences, has numerous publications to her credit, and has funded her research efforts consistently since 1995. She has mentored countless graduate and undergraduate students, introducing them to research and careers in psychiatric and gerontological nursing. She lives in Miami with her husband Francis Henderson.

Carol Davis, PT, EdD, MS, FAPTA, has practiced physical therapy for over 30 years, beginning her career at the Massachusetts General Hospital in 1969. She completed her Doctorate in Humanistic Studies at Boston University in 1982, and has been on the faculty at the University of Miami since that time, except for a 2.5-year position at Boston University from 1985 to 1987. Currently, she is a tenured professor in the Department of Physical Therapy at the University of Miami School of Medicine. She is the author of *Complementary Therapies in Rehabilitation: Evidence for Efficacy in Therapy, Prevention, and Wellness, Second Edition;* three editions of *Patient Practitioner Interaction: An Experiential Manual for Developing the Art of Health Care;* and a videotape lecture entitled *The Challenge of the New Millennium—Returning Healing to Health Care: Theoretical Foundation of Holistic Complementary Therapies.* She has also presented many papers nationally and internationally.

CONTRIBUTING AUTHORS

Lois S. Marshall, PhD, RN, CPN
Wallace Gilroy Endowed Chair in Nursing
Associate Professor of Clinical Nursing
Associate Dean for Undergraduate Studies
School of Nursing
University of Miami
Coral Gables, Fla

Tamika R. Sanchez-Jones, RN, C, MBA, PhD(c)
Doctoral Candidate
School of Nursing
University of Miami
Coral Gables, Fla

Nancy E. Villanueva, PhD, ARNP, BC, CNRN
Nurse Practitioner, Neurosurgery
Jackson Memorial Hospital
Miami, Fla

FOREWORD

Therapeutic Interaction in Nursing is a compendium of superb content dealing with communication of nurses with a wide variety of clients. But significantly, while written with a student nurse audience in mind, the authors provide information that is suitable for the spectrum of health professionals—students and practitioners alike. Perhaps the learning tools provided will be more or less used depending on the level of the practitioner, but they are all sound and can be used with personal discretion.

Communication is the *sine qua non* of therapeutic interactions with patients. Communication has been getting new attention in other health disciplines, such as medicine, but has been part of nursing's educational regime for many decades. Either as separate courses or as modules within other courses, nursing educators have shown their realization that understanding the meaning of communication and communication strategies are vital to the practice of nursing.

This book is extremely impressive in both the currency of the references and the delving back into the literature so that we are not bombarded with the new while ignoring the major thinkers in the field whose work laid the basis for the newer theorists. This is to be applauded. Too many writers today are familiar with current thinking but go back so few years that the depth of their content has the feeling of "born yesterday." This is definitely not the case with Williams and Davis.

The first chapter on understanding one's self exemplifies this characteristic of the thoughtful work of the authors. Starting with the essentials of understanding one's self, Williams and Davis explore the latest theories with regard to intelligence. However, the interpersonal theory of psychiatry, which presages much of the recent thinking, is explored as well. This chapter is a must for every reader.

The second and third chapters, which explore the helping relationship, are basic to understanding the chapter on communication strategies that follows. Thorough exploration of the concept of helping focuses on the interpersonal relationship of nurse and client and terms it a collaboration. Starting with this concept, the authors then define terms that will be used over and over again in the young professionals' lives and should become second nature to them as they seek to understand their own and clients' reactions and interactions.

In the fourth chapter, the health care encounter—the interview itself—is described in a way that can be used for independent study as well as classroom study with an instructor. I can see myself using this chapter in both classroom teaching and in observing a student using the strategies delineated in the chapter. It is an excellent guide for both student and teacher.

Sanchez-Jones writes with sensitivity and great knowledge about communicating across cultures. This very valuable chapter can stand on its own for professionals who feel quite confident with audiences similar to themselves but less so with people who are different.

The remainder of the book deals with communication with specific groups of patients. Again, the sensitivity with which these subjects is handled is commendable and makes for very good reading. While some of these areas will be useful for reference again and again as nurses are dealing with special populations, they are intellectually stimulating even without such contacts.

This book fills a gap in the field and should be extremely useful in curricula, regardless of the method of teaching this important subject. I would recommend its use in both discrete courses and modules in communication as well as in courses dealing with the specialized subject matter discussed in the second half of the book.

Claire M. Fagin, PhD, RN, FAAN
Dean Emerita, Professor Emerita
University of Pennsylvania
School of Nursing
Philadelphia, Pa
Director, John A. Hartford Foundation Building Academic Geriatric Capacity Scholars Program

INTRODUCTION

In choosing the title for this book I intended to convey two messages. In the word *therapeutic* I mean healing. To heal is to foster wholeness or integration of mind, body, and spirit. Each component of the person is recognized and valued. The second word in the title is *interaction,* which connotes taking action or playing an active role in each opportunity to be with clients. Each encounter between nurse and client, whether brief or extended, is an opportunity for healing. The nurse takes responsibility for engaging the client in an experience that enhances wholeness and well-being.

I was motivated to write this book because I have taught this subject to students and practicing nurses for 28 years and have found insufficient information in print. It has been my experience that students need further explanation than the material found in textbooks designed to integrate communication topics along with many other concepts. Over the years I have developed numerous supplementary materials to enhance student learning about the nature and importance of nurse-client communication, and this book offers an opportunity to consolidate these materials and to apply current knowledge to specialized clinical situations such as communication with individuals with cognitive impairment.

The idea for *Therapeutic Interaction in Nursing* was conceived when I was approached by Carol Davis. Carol and I had worked together at the University of Miami for several years on interdisciplinary projects including the Executive Committee of the Miami Area Geriatric Education Center (MAGEC) and the Geriatric Interdisciplinary Faculty Team (GIFT). Carol's book *Patient Practitioner Interaction* (PPI), a book about communication for physical therapists, was in the third edition (and a fourth edition is in process) and we discussed writing a book about communication specifically directed toward nurses. With this conversation, *Therapeutic Interaction in Nursing* began to take shape. I would like to acknowledge Carol for her unique insights into professional relationships and communication for health care professionals. She has been extremely helpful throughout the writing of this book and her support was invaluable to me.

This book is ideal for a course in communication for nurses. It will also be invaluable as a text in an integrated nursing program. The introductory chapters and companion exercises in Sections I and II will enhance learning in early clinical courses. The chapters in Section III dealing with specific clinical groups can be assigned when students are engaged in those clinical experiences.

The information contained in Sections I and II can be used by any nurse preparing for certification or licensure examinations. This information is essential for advanced practice nurses and health professionals. The discussion of special topics contained in the section Communicating in Special Circumstances will be a useful resource for clinicians and graduate students who are working with special populations.

Christine L. Williams, DNSc, RN, BC

Therapeutic Use
of Self

Understanding the Self

Carol M. Davis, PT, EdD, MS, FAPTA and Christine L. Williams, DNSc, RN, BC

OBJECTIVES

1. To discuss the importance of self-awareness to effective helping
2. To examine the development of a mature person as described by Erikson
3. To describe the role of childhood development in the formation of identity and self-esteem

It has been said that a nurse's most important tool is the therapeutic use of self. Therapeutic use of self means nurses employing their emotions and perceptions to understand clients' health needs and their knowledge and skills to facilitate the healing process. Our personalities and styles of relating have everything to do with how effectively we facilitate the healing process. If we were to ask nurses to assess their ability to relate effectively with people, few would admit to lapses in temper, irritability, or prejudice. Yet, these and other negative behaviors can occur, especially when nurses lack self-awareness.

Although difficult to observe, behaviors such as lack of honesty and loyalty to one's colleagues and breaking confidences are common in health care. Often, nurses are unaware of their unprofessional behavior or the effect of their behavior on others. Clients challenge our sensitivity and maturity in unique ways. Clients react out of the stress of their illnesses or pain, but nurses must also work under stress. It requires great maturity and patience to respond in healing ways in less than ideal situations.

EMOTIONAL INTELLIGENCE

Since intelligence is multidimensional, cognitive or thinking intelligence is not enough to ensure that a nurse will be effective with patients. Another type of intelligence is necessary as well: emotional intelligence.[1] Emotional intelligence is the ability to understand one's emotions and to use those emotions effectively in social situations.[2] The nurse who can choose where, when, and how to express his or her emotions will avoid impulsive expression of potentially destructive emotions such as anger. Such self-control is essential to therapeutic interaction.

Emotional intelligence is important in another component of therapeutic interaction: the ability to understand emotions in others. Responding with compassion is possible when the nurse can see the hurt in an angry client's outburst or the fear in individuals who delay treatment until their condition becomes life-threatening. Understanding the emotions that trigger behavior is fundamental to appreciating and caring for clients.[1]

Emotions cannot be separated from their neurobiological basis. LeDoux writes that there are two pathways from perceiving threat to action. One is a direct route through the emotional center of the brain, the amygdala. This kind of reaction is immediate and results in behavior on an emotional level without much thought. The other route is through the neocortex, the thinking part of the brain, where emotions are considered along with knowledge and experience. This slower, more thoughtful approach is likely to lead to rational behavior. When faced with a threat, the individual may react without thinking and come to regret those actions later. Therapeutic communication depends on the nurse's ability to react with thought as well as emotion in order to handle emotionally charged situations in a rational way.[3]

INFLUENCE OF THE FAMILY ON SELF-ESTEEM

Each of us views the world from a unique perspective. We begin to develop our unique perspective as small children. Our worldview evolves out of what we hear and experience as children growing up in a unique family unit. Children are influenced by their parents' view of the world. Other important adults, such as close relatives and teachers, provide another important source of guidance. We develop our sense of self through interactions with parents or caregivers.[4] These important people guide children with tenderness when their behavior meets with their approval or redirect behaviors that fail to meet expectations. These learning experiences, combined with inborn characteristics, develop into a unique way of experiencing the world. Even twins growing up under the same circumstances will develop different views based upon which each chooses to notice.

Children are not little adults, as Piaget first clearly described.[5] Children have underdeveloped nervous systems and lack the capacity to move, think, and act in the same manner as adults. Children live in a land of make believe, enjoy fantasy, and are egocentric. They are unable to handle abstract logic and are very present oriented and concrete. If you ask a child which of two parallel, identical pencils is longer, she or he will say, correctly, that both are the same length. But then if you slide one pencil so that it is ahead of the other, though still parallel, and then ask, "Which pencil is longer?" she or he will say the pen-

cil that is ahead of the other is longer. In other words, children cannot conserve information. Likewise, children are unable to come outside of themselves and view themselves. Ask a child who has a brother if he has a brother and he'll say "Yes." Ask him if his brother has a brother, he'll say "No."[6]

Finally, children idolize their parents. They cope with feelings of helplessness and dependence by believing that their parents (or caregivers) are powerful and will protect them and care for them. Even when parents fail to protect them or meet their needs, most children continue to believe in them and will deny the negative experiences of the past.

> **Case Example**
> Samuel experienced severe neglect from his mother, Claire, during his early years. When he was 10 years of age, they were separated for 6 months except for occasional supervised visits while Claire was treated for substance abuse in a long-term drug rehabilitation program. He was cared for by loving and attentive relatives. During the separation, he longed to be returned to his mother and looked forward to her visits with great excitement. He never referred to his suffering during those early years and seemed to remember only positive memories.

Erik Erikson[7] developed a useful description of the development of personality that centers on the successful resolution of tension in a series of steps encountered by the growing person from birth onward. A certain degree of accomplishment is required at each stage or the child will have to master those tasks later in life. Table 1-1 summarizes Erikson's theory of development.

Human beings are among few living creatures born without the capacity to crawl, wiggle, or walk to a source of food. It might be said that we are 9 months in the womb and 9 (or more) months out, totally helpless to move about to a source of food or nourishment. As infants, we must cry out to others around us in order to have our basic survival needs met. The fact that we are born totally dependent on others for our survival is a critical aspect of the development of our worldview. Who we are and our perceptions of the world depend on how others respond to us when we are helpless and on what others say to us and about us. This is how our identity develops. It

Table 1-1

PSYCHOSOCIAL THEORY OF DEVELOPMENT:
A SUMMARY OF ERIKSON'S EPIGENETIC STAGES OF DEVELOPMENT

Trust vs Mistrust (0 to 12 Months)

From birth to approximately 1 year, this stage is the basis for all future development of personality. A feeling of physical comfort accompanied by minimal fear and uncertainty results in an infant's sense of trust. The quality of the relationship with mother or maternal figure is more important than quantity of food or demonstrations of love. Experiences with one's body are the first and primary means of social interactions for the baby, thus they provide the foundations for psychological trust. The issues involved in trust and mistrust are not settled for all time during this phase of life; they may arise again and again during development and later life. Later confrontation with trust may shake one's basic trust or provide another opportunity for further development if these needs were not adequately met the first time.

Autonomy vs Shame and Doubt (2 to 4 Years)

As the child of 2 to 4 years experiences the world around him, he begins to discover that his behavior can bring about certain results. Out of these encounters with reality grows a sense of autonomy. At the same time, the child has some conflicts about asserting or remaining dependent in different types of situations. Exploring is a primary goal of this growing and increasingly coordinated physical being. It becomes more and more difficult to remain in a confined place. The child is occupied with activities involving retaining and releasing—manipulating objects, expressing himself, making new friends and letting them go, and bodily functions. The degree to which the child will allow others to regulate his behavior is regularly tested, leading to a greater sense of self-understanding and responsibility or, in the case of over-control, leading to shame and doubt.

Initiative vs Guilt (4 to 5 Years)

During the fourth and fifth years, language development and locomotion have reached a sufficiently high level to permit expansion of imagination. Play activities are more interesting and companionship with peers is sought. There is curiosity and comparison with others around size and skill issues—who is the better tree climber, who is biggest or best at almost anything. The child in this stage is into everything and seeks attention verbally and physically. Sexual curiosity and genital stimulation are apparent. Adult treatment of the curiosity will reinforce the initiative or result in shame and guilt. Because of a very active imagination, the child may feel guilty for sexual thoughts and for activities that no one has observed. The evolving conscience is becoming established and will ultimately control initiative. If the child's activities are perceived as a nuisance, whether motor or verbal, she may develop feelings of guilt over self-initiated activities, which may last a lifetime. Healthy identification with parents, teachers, and peers helps resolve some of the guilt problems.

Industry vs Inferiority (6 to 11 Years)

Between the ages of 6 and 11 the child moves seriously into the world of competition and the separation of work and play. The individuals having impact on this developing sense of self now include many other adults and a wider sphere of peers. As the lessons of work are learned, the child often needs to slip into the familiar play world to bolster what may feel like flagging initiative. The developing industry evolves from efforts and achievements rewarded by significant others and leads to a sense of social worth. When the child learns social worth is linked to background of parents, color of skin, or the label on his clothes, identity with those conditions rather than self may result. These first four stages form the base upon which the adolescent builds a sense of identity.

Identity vs Identity Diffusion (12 to 18 Years)

During this stage of changes, the consistent task is striving to be oneself and to share oneself with something else. The beginning of separation from parents finally becomes a serious agenda. The adolescent experiences the need to be master of her own affairs and free of dependency. The emerging young adult is eager to know her abilities and to have the adult world recognize them as well. The adolescent also fears that the demands of adulthood will exceed the capacities to meet them. Time perspective vs time diffusion becomes the dilemma. When the adult world offers the adolescent responsibilities and privileges at an appropriate pace (com-

---

Table 1-1 (continued)

PSYCHOSOCIAL THEORY OF DEVELOPMENT: A SUMMARY OF ERIKSON'S EPIGENETIC STAGES OF DEVELOPMENT

mensurate with capacity and desires), there is resolution of some of the issues with a sense of time perspective, as opposed to urgency and hopelessness. The derivatives of the second stage of "autonomy vs shame and doubt" are reworked in the adolescent in the form of establishing a sense of self-certainty. When adults can offer reinforcement appropriately to build the adolescent's self-esteem, feelings of inferiority diminish. The remains of "initiative vs guilt" reappear with the need to discover individualized and unique talents and interests. There seems to be a need to experiment with different roles and express initiative in different ways. If stymied in this dimension, it may seem easier to resolve the conflict by seeking behavior or roles in conflict with parents or the community, thus achieving a negative identity that is preferable to an "identity diffusion," which is experienced as being nobody at all. Most authorities agree that the period of adolescence brings with it an increase in psychic energy. The young person who uses these energies effectively can experiment in many ways and have experiences of achievement. If much of the energy is used to resolve feelings resulting from earlier unresolved crises, which often reappear at this time, then the rather fragile sense of self may be seriously threatened, with introspection interfering with concentration. The successful resolution of adolescent tasks and the development of a strong sense of identity may require many years beyond age 18. During this time, the young adult experiments with new behavior and may ignore some societal mores in the process. It is important for this process to work itself through, especially with talented and creative persons. Negative labeling may reinforce a temporary identity which, given time, will work itself into something else.

Intimacy vs Isolation (Young Adulthood)

The first phase of adulthood comes into being after the adolescent has worked out a sense of identity. Sexual and psychological intimacies between two people while retaining one's own identity is the primary task of this stage. This goal is sought through forms of friendship, leadership, athletics, even combat. Unwillingness or inability to achieve intimacy will result in distancing oneself from others who pose a threat to identity. Achievement is characterized by the ability and willingness to share with another in mutual trust, to regulate cycles of work, and to participate in society in self-satisfying ways. This stage continues through early middle age.

Generativity vs Stagnation (Middle Adulthood)

The basic agenda of the middle years is aimed at guiding the next generation, whether in parenting or through employment and enjoyment situations. The critical question of this time occurs when the individual looks back to examine what has happened up to that time in life and whether it was satisfying. If the individual turns inward and becomes self-absorbed, stagnation results.

Integrity vs Despair (Older Adulthood)

The primary task of the later years is the acceptance of oneself and one's life. When the individual has experienced the feelings that accompany a share of the good things of life without being overwhelmed by its tragedies, disappointments, and frustrations, ego integrity is the result. There is acceptance of one's existence with full responsibility and commitment to a certain way of life and its values. Having experienced what is felt to be a full life, the individual can accept giving it up with "integrity." If, on the other hand, the person feels there has been little good from life and there are few prospects of any good coming, there is a sense of despair often accompanied by fear of death.

Reprinted with permission from Ramsden E. Affective dimensions in client care. In: Payton O, ed. *Psychosocial Aspects of Clinical Practice.* New York: Churchill Livingstone; 1986.

is obvious that the maturity of the parent and the extent to which the child is wanted and anticipated have a great deal to do with how the parent responds to the child and thus fosters or inhibits the development of a sense of self-identity and self-esteem.

Few of us grew up in ideal homes, but many of us have difficulty remembering the negative things about childhood. Remember that children idealize their parents. Adolescents give up those notions, but many replace them with strongly held traditions to honor and respect their parents. To idealize your parents is to idealize the way they raised you.[8] Part of maturation is to give up the idealized view of our parents and to replace it with a balanced awareness of their strengths and weaknesses. It is very important to look back at what was happening in your family when you were growing up as one way to increase your awareness of your self and your worldview.

Each child is born into a complex family situation and encounters various challenges, as described by Erikson, as he or she develops day-by-day. If a child is born to parents who experience physical comfort, emotional calm, and joy in his or her presence, the child will develop a sense of trust and a view that the world is a warm and loving place. If, however, the child is a burden to parents, he or she will come to believe that the world is uncertain. A child born to a family with violent parents will experience the world as a hostile place and will learn to mistrust others. In fact, painful childhood memories are stored in the brain even when we have limited ability to describe them in words. These memories continue to affect our behavior as adults until we become more aware of them and replace them with positive experiences.[1]

It is unrealistic to expect a child to complete each stage of development on schedule without any difficulties. Children may have partial resolution of a developmental task at times or may be unsuccessful at other times. The degree of success with a stage of development will influence the child's ability to successfully complete the next stage. Adults may still be working on developmental tasks from childhood because they were unable to complete them successfully at the time. Parents use their own experience to guide their children through these tasks. Generally, adults who do not parent well were not parented well themselves. Dysfunctional parents learn to be dysfunctional from the families in which they grew up.

Case Example

Sara is the 22-year-old mother of 18-month-old Cami. Cami is a healthy, active toddler who loves to run and is unaware of dangerous situations in the environment. Sara enjoys taking Cami to the park where she meets other young mothers with their children. Sara's ideas about parenting are based on the way she was parented. She expects Cami to obey her when she commands her to "Stop running!" or to come to her when she calls her name. When Cami looks back at her mother, laughs, and keeps running, Sara is enraged and slaps her to communicate her disapproval. Sara cannot understand why her daughter continues to "disobey," and Cami cannot understand why her mother withdraws her approval. Cami is learning to be distrustful and doubtful about her growing independence.

How we respond to the world today is influenced by our biological attributes, past experiences, sense of ourselves, and the adequacy of our self-esteem. The development of healthy self-esteem requires more successful than unsuccessful resolution of the tensions described by Erikson either as we mature or later. As adults, we can examine our growing up experiences, gain insight into our dysfunctional views, and consciously change our distorted worldview to give us a more accurate focus of the world and of ourselves.

HEALTHY OR OPEN FAMILIES

Healthy families interact in ways that have been described as "open" in contrast to the "closed" functioning of troubled or dysfunctional families (Table 1-2). A family functions to provide a safe and supportive environment for all of its members to learn basic values, to grow, and to become more fully human. In healthy families, members feel empowered to adapt to change and supported in coping with the stresses of the world both outside the home and within. The stress inside the home is usually perceived to be less than the stress faced outside in the world, except in transient phases of family crisis.

Table 1-2

CHARACTERISTICS OF FAMILIES

Open/Healthy	Troubled	Closed/Unhealthy
Open to change	Nothing can be done	Rigid, fixed, harsh rules
Flexible responses to each situation	What's the use?	Right vs wrong, no exceptions
High self-worth	Shaky self-worth	Evasive responses
People are valued as individuals	Hides feelings of low self-control	Low self-worth, shaming behavior Low ownership—blaming
Functional defenses Use defenses as a coping skill with insight	Use defenses to hide pain Defenses more often deny real feelings Choice is lost Always smile, cry, or complain	No choice—react compulsively and rigidly out of fear Short fuses Avoidance of rage
Clear rules discussed: hours, respect for property, telephone use, chores, etc Rules are regularly negotiated	Unclear—rules are inconsistent Depends on who is asked, what day, which child	Edicts or no rules at all Chaos—rules cannot be followed
People take risks to express feelings, ideas, beliefs	Not safe to express feelings or give opinions: "Don't rock the boat" Can't disagree	Denial of problems Ignore bizarre behaviors No talk rule—even about serious problems, especially drinking, drugs
Can deal with stress, pick up on other's pain Nurturing and caring for each other Seek out those in pain to support, encourage	Avoid pain Do not see it in others Sweep problems under the rug Pretend all is okay	Denial of stress Cannot cope with any more—glazed eyes do not see pain Ignore basic need to be seen, acknowledged Children become early helpers
Accepts life stages, welcomes them Celebrate growth—sexuality, new friends, accomplishments	Parents may compete with children—growth is accepted painfully—do not talk about sex Try to keep children dependent	Passage of time is ignored Change is feared—adults are treated as children, children may try to act like adults Children are ridiculed, teased, but try to become helpful

Table 1-2 (continued)

CHARACTERISTICS OF FAMILIES

Open/Healthy	Troubled	Closed/Unhealthy
Either clear hierarchy or egalitarian—strong parental coalition	Hidden coalitions across generations	Either upside down family—children may run it—or chaotic
Less need to control	Parental coalition is weak— rigid or shifting pattern of domination	No giving out of rules, or one parent is in charge of all and cannot cope
Can negotiate		
Affect is open	Negativism, low feeling, bickering, argumentative, controlled mood, some feelings are okay, some not	Cynicism, open hostility, violence, sadism—actually try to manipulate and hurt each other
Direct expression of feelings, all feelings are okay	Inconsistent acceptance of feelings	Only happiness is allowed
Anger is in context of awareness of other person		
Considerate of others		

Reprinted with permission from Davis CM. *Patient Practitioner Interaction: An Experiential Manual for Developing the Art of Health Care*. 3rd Ed. Thorofare, NJ: SLACK Incorporated; 1998.

Individuals are recognized as being unique and having worth. There is value to the family unit, and there is open communication in which members feel free to speak their opinion but do so with concern and caring for others. In sum, family members feel safe, supported, encouraged, and appreciated. Roles and responsibilities of family members are flexible but clear. People function well day-to-day and in crisis. Finally, quality time is shared by parents and children and is enjoyed.[9]

DYSFUNCTIONAL OR CLOSED FAMILIES

Charles Whitfield believes that many people grow up in families that stifle the development of the true self and instead cultivate in the child a false or "codependent" self.[10] Children need to feel as if they are safe and protected at all times. They need to feel free to ask questions, to run and play, to know the boundaries that parents set for them are fair and consistent. Children need to feel as if they can be children, learning and growing without fear of being ridiculed or punished cruelly for making mistakes. Children need to be invited to feel their feelings and put them into words so that they can learn gently how not to be impulsive and controlled by their feelings.

Dysfunctional families, however, respond to the dependence of a child in ways that interfere with the development of authenticity. In the dysfunctional family, children do not feel free to make mistakes, but feel that if they are not "right" they will be harshly criticized. In such a family, children receive approval when they are compliant, considerate, and unselfish.[10] Adults assume the role of authoritarian masters, intent on breaking the child's will at any cost, or they tend to absent themselves totally from parenting, escaping in alcohol, work, mental illness, or travel. Children, who think of their parents as perfect, soon begin realizing that they are not free to act natural or to be a child. They may adopt another way of being, usually that of comforting and nurturing the parent. The child thus becomes parent to the parent. As a result, a false self emerges in the child. According to psychologist Alice Miller,[11] the persistent denial of the true self and true feelings takes its toll in the development of coping mechanisms and a realistic view of the world.

HEALTH PROFESSIONALS' SELF-ESTEEM

It has been said that many people enter the health professions for a variety of reasons. Among those reasons might be a need to be depended upon, a need to control people, and a need to get one's natural attention and affection needs met. Some may be looking for emotional healing themselves by way of making life easier for others. Few people are conscious of these motives, however. Nonetheless, some health professionals act in ways that are responsive to their emotions and do things that are, in the long run, harmful to clients and contrary to the healing process. These are the characteristics of *early helpers*.

Dysfunctional families often create children who can be described as early helpers. One example of a dysfunctional family is that in which one or both parents are addicted to alcohol. Millions of Americans grew up or are presently living with an alcoholic.[12] The literature that has developed from the Adult Children of Alcoholics (ACOA) movement in the United States has shed needed light on the distorted worldview of the adult who grew up in a home in which one or more parents were unable or unwilling to parent. This circumstance encourages the development of the "false self," stifles the successful resolution of the tensions described by Erikson, and contributes to chronic low self-esteem and feelings of not being "good enough."[9] All children experience shame, but children in dysfunctional families take on shame as part of their identity. Children in dysfunctional families are never free to be children; they have to be grown-up and helpful. Since this is indeed a difficult task, they feel that they are always doing something wrong. Shame is different from guilt. Whitfield[10] describes shame as "the uncomfortable or painful feeling that we experience when we realize that part of us is defective, bad, incomplete, rotten, phony, inadequate, or a failure." Thus, guilt says, "I made a mistake"; shame says, "I am a mistake."

Self-esteem can be viewed as the extent to which we are able and willing to believe in our essential goodness in the face of our own lack of perfection. More than simply self-acceptance, self-esteem includes pride in the promise of ongoing growth and change with maturity, the hope of a richer, more peaceful and congruent life as a result of honest, day-to-day struggle. Children reared in dysfunctional families feel the shame of never being quite good enough rather than confidence and pride in doing the best they can. When feelings of shame are identified and replaced with a more realistic view of our imperfections and essential goodness, self-acceptance becomes possible.

Parental dysfunction may result from many causes. The critical factor seems to be how well the parent was present for the growing child in such a way as to encourage the natural curiosity of the child; the natural desire to learn, grow, and explore the world; how well the parent nurtured and protected the child; and how safe and free from potential harm the child felt.[10] When the parent absents him- or herself from those responsibilities, for whatever reason (drug dependence, workaholism, depression or mental illness, absence of a good model for parenting), the child starts parenting the parent, and an early helper emerges. A common description given by children from dysfunctional families is that they feel that they were a burden; they feel that they were being bad when they simply showed natural curiosity or asked questions. In fact, it was their very existence that seemed to bring discomfort to their family.[10]

Children are not meant to be parents. When they take on this role, they take on a false self, and authentic feelings of curiosity, fear, and need become repressed, covered by feigned feelings of bravery and affection in an attempt to please the parent. Common characteristics that materialize from the distorted worldview and false view of the self include:

* Fear of losing control
* Fear of feelings that seem overwhelming
* Fear of conflict
* Fear of abandonment
* Fear of becoming alcoholic or drug dependent
* Fear of becoming dependent on another person for survival
* Overdeveloped sense of responsibility
* Feelings of guilt and grief
* Inability to relax and have fun spontaneously
* Harsh self-criticism
* A tendency to lie, even when the truth would have been readily accepted
* A tendency to let one's mind wander, to lose track of a conversation, to figuratively "leave the room." Denial and/or the tendency to create reality the way you want it to be, rather than the way it is
* Difficulties getting close to people, difficulties with intimacy
* Feelings of vulnerability, of being a victim in a harsh world

* Compulsive behavior, tendency to become addicted to things that alter mood
* Comfort with taking charge in a crisis; panic if you cannot "do" something in a crisis
* Confusion between love and pity
* Black and white perspective—all good or all bad
* Internalizing—taking responsibility for others' problems
* Tendency to react rather than act
* Experiencing stress-related illnesses
* Overachievement

Children from dysfunctional families are the "heroes" in health care, the ones who, at great personal sacrifice, go above and beyond the call to fix things for everyone else and are praised and admired for it. They thrive on rescuing others and on creating order out of chaos. Very often, these are the people whom others admonish to "lighten up," for they take every aspect of their lives very seriously.

THE NEED TO KNOW OURSELVES

The nurse must know him- or herself well; he or she must be aware of behaviors that will result in harmful dependence on clients for meeting personal needs for intimacy. The end goal of all healing is the restoration of independent function for the highest and deepest quality of life possible for the client. Clients who depend on us for this function never feel able to make it on their own. We foster this destructive dependence when we, ourselves, depend on our clients to meet our needs for attention, affection, and/or power and authority.

Self-awareness helps us to identify our emotions and to monitor our own behavior. It is very difficult to help others if we need help ourselves. Help is widely available through counseling, participation in support groups and psychotherapy groups, and in 12-step programs such as Al Anon, Overeaters Anonymous, Alcoholics Anonymous, and Adult Children of Alcoholics (ACOA), all of which can be found throughout the United States and in other countries. The goal of seeking help is always to become acquainted with the true self and to gain self-acceptance.

CONCLUSION

A lack of self-understanding can interfere with helping others; therefore, taking the time to reflect on your past as well as your present life is a crucial part of a career in nursing. Becoming familiar with your strengths and vulnerabilities will help you to minimize inappropriate emotional reactions and maximize thoughtful, compassionate responses to the needs of clients. Developing self-understanding and learning to use your emotions to enhance relationships will be a lifelong process. Caring for people of different backgrounds and in a variety of life experiences will forever challenge you to grow personally.

REFERENCES

1. Goleman D. *Emotional Intelligence*. New York: Bantam Books; 1995.
2. Schutte NS, Malouff, JM, Bobik C. Emotional intelligence and interpersonal relations. *The Journal of Social Psychology*. 2001;141(4):523-536.
3. LeDoux J. *The Emotional Brain*. New York: Touchstone; 1996.
4. Sullivan HS. *The Interpersonal Theory of Psychiatry*. New York: WW Norton & Company; 1954.
5. Piaget J. *The Construction of Reality in the Child*. New York: Basic Books; 1954.
6. Bradshaw J. *Bradshaw on: The Family*. Deerfield Beach, Fla: Health Communications, Inc; 1988.
7. Erikson EH. *Identity, Youth and Crisis*. New York: WW Norton; 1968.
8. Rogers CR. *On Becoming a Person*. Boston: Houghton Miflin Company; 1961.
9. *Identifying Successful Families: An Overview of Constructs and Selected Resources*. Washington, DC: Department of Health and Human Services; 1990.
10. Whitfield CL. *Healing the Child Within*. Baltimore: The Resource Group; 1986.
11. Miller A. *The Drama of the Gifted Child*. New York: Basic Books; 1981.
12. Grant BF. Prevalence and correlates of alcohol use and DSM-IV alcohol dependence in the United States: results of the National Longitudinal Alcohol Epidemiologic Survey. *Journal of Studies on Alcohol*. 1997;58(5):464-473.

EXERCISES

1. Self-Assessment

In a spiral notebook that you can keep confidential, answer each of the following questions as honestly as you can for this moment. It is suggested that you use a notebook so that you can save these reflections and refer back to them later. Allow at least half a page for each question. Jot down the first thing that comes to mind for each question, then take additional time to express your thoughts clearly. You may wish to complete the entire set over a period of a week or so, taking one or two questions at a time. When you have completed these exercises, share your conclusions with a trusted friend or confidant.

A. Who am I?

Date:

* I would describe myself physically as...

* I would describe my personality as...

* Others would describe me as...

* When I think about who I am, I am most proud of...

* I was most ashamed of...

* I get angriest when...

* I am most anxious that...

* When I am nervous I usually...

* People are essentially (good, bad, neutral)...

* Characteristics of other people that impress me most include...

* Goals I want to achieve:

    With this course...

    In my lifetime...

Discussion

Once you have answered these questions, write a description about yourself from what you have discovered. Are you totally happy with yourself at this point? What would you change? What did you learn about yourself that will assist you in being a health professional? What may detract from your effectiveness?

B. What about my family of origin (those who raised me)?

✳ If I were to use one word to describe my family (as a whole) it would be...

✳ The best thing about growing up in my family was...

✳ The most challenging part of growing up in my family was...

✳ In my family, disagreements were...

✳ In my family, talking about a problem was...

Discussion

When you have answered these questions, summarize what you have learned about your family of origin. How have you learned to relate to others? In what ways will your experiences affect how you relate with clients?

2. Journal

In your self-assessment notebook, begin a journal about yourself. Most of us confuse the concept of a journal with a diary. A diary is designed to record significant events in one's life. A journal is a letter to yourself, designed to stimulate reflection about an experience rather than just recording the experience. One way to keep from simply recording the event is to begin each entry with the following phrases:

✳ What I felt during the exercise.

✳ What I learned about myself.

✳ So what? Significance or meanings of my learning.

Your journal should be kept in a book with a cover, on pages that do not easily become dislodged. Entries are to be written following each chapter. Many find it useful to journal as a way of privately discussing the chapter and its personal significance. Your journal is what you make it. Most university students are unaccustomed to this sort of activity, however, and some abhor writing. For a short time, make a commitment to this activity. Remember, this journal is by you, for your personal use. Set aside the time on your calendar and once you get into the routine of it, it will become rewarding. Your course instructor may wish to see your entries now and again to be sure you are keeping up. In that case, confidentiality may become more limited. **You will not be graded on your journal.** Since it is a collection of your feelings and reflections, a grade would be wholly inappropriate. However, the value of the activity is such that your instructor may collect it to check your discipline with the activity and may comment on how well you reflected on the experience rather than simply describing what happened.

3. Family Genogram

A genogram is a map of a family for several generations. It is a very useful picture that reveals patterns. An example of a genogram is shown below. Different symbols are used to represent male and female members of the family as well as type and quality of the relationships.

Draw a diagram of your family—your family genogram—for at least three generations. Label anything that seems important to you. A genogram is a way to display relationships within a family across generations.

What patterns emerge? What do you now know about yourself that you failed to see before? What stories are important enough to be handed down? Who/what is the family proud of? What secrets does the family hide from others?

Perhaps questions came up for you about various family members' lives and habits. Write to relatives asking them to fill in the missing pieces to help you better understand your heritage. Try to locate pictures from long ago of yourself with other family members.

Journal about your feelings and awareness from this exercise. Can you identify behaviors that you have developed from your family that may interfere with helping others? Comment on any and problem solve ways in which you might be able to work through those behaviors.

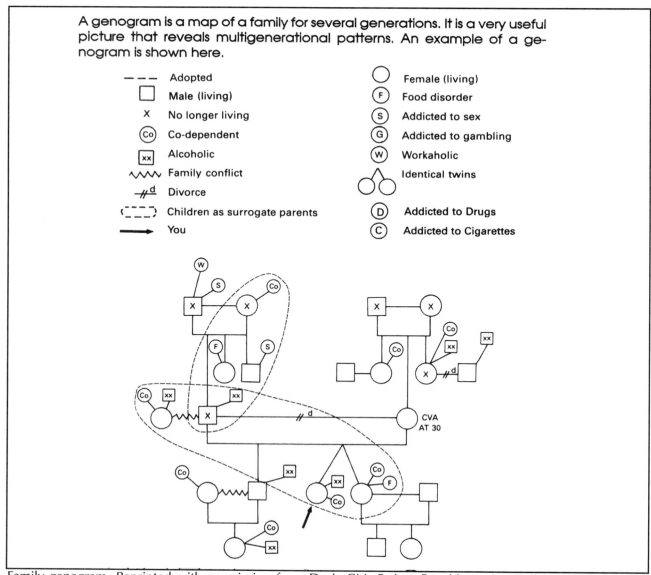

Family genogram. Reprinted with permission from Davis CM. *Patient Practitioner Interaction: An Experiential Manual for Developing the Art of Health Care.* 3rd Ed. Thorofare, NJ: SLACK Incorporated; 1998.

Using the Self to Promote Health

Carol M. Davis, PT, EdD, MS, FAPTA and Christine L. Williams, DNSc, RN, BC

OBJECTIVES

1. To consider the overall aim of helping
2. To explore the behaviors that interfere with effective helping
3. To describe some of the characteristics of helping communication
4. To distinguish empathy from related interpersonal interactions
5. To reveal the characteristics of effective helpers

What should be the overall aim of helping? Infants who need help rely on others to make them feel better. As young children, we often lack the skills to solve our own problems, so we depend on some capable adult to take charge. Unlike children, adults require a different sort of helping. Balancing self-reliance with the ability to ask for help strengthens an adult's confidence and self-esteem. When the nurse relies on giving advice, the client may become resentful and angry and feel helpless and dependent. When the nurse has a need to be told how helpful or even how irreplaceable he or she is to the client, the client's needs become secondary and the nurse loses effectiveness.

No person can take responsibility for another person. We can only take responsibility for ourselves. The overall aim of helping is to assist the client in becoming self-sufficient and achieving a more effective relationship between self and others. Clients may come to us with or without a diagnosis, but the key questions remain: What are the health issues from the client's perspective? And what are the client's goals in the healing process? Exceptions are children and adults who have lost the ability to be adequately in charge of their own lives—those with certain mental illnesses and those with brain dysfunction. Even then, we consider the perspective of the family.

Hildegard Peplau,[1] the "mother of psychiatric nursing," wrote that "nursing is a human relationship between an individual who is sick or in need of health services and a nurse especially educated to recognize and to respond to the need for help." The help that nurses offer to their clients is much more than technical expertise. The relationship between nurse and client is a powerful healing force by itself. Peplau also wrote that nursing is both educative and therapeutic. Every interaction between a nurse and a client includes a learning experience for the client about relationships, helping relationships in particular. If the client experiences a collaborative relationship with the nurse in which he or she is accepted and valued, the result will be personal growth and development. The client will be strengthened and better able to meet similar crises in the future.

_...ctive helping involves identifying opportunities for growth as well as problems. As nurses, we learn important knowledge, skills, and values that we offer to assist clients who need help to understand their health and to act in ways that promote health. We provide the conditions for our clients to identify their goals and then help them to meet those goals.

Therapeutic communication, or the use of verbal and nonverbal messages to establish a therapeutic relationship, is also essential to the use of the self as an instrument of healing. Therapeutic communication will be explained in greater detail in this chapter and throughout this book.

How you view yourself will markedly affect your communication with clients. Remember that your self-concept affects the way you view the world and the way you communicate. Most of us have felt the discomfort of interacting with a person who continually apologizes for him- or herself, who distorts what we say, or who responds with negativity and self-contempt. Each of us holds opinions and ideas about ourselves, but our essential self-worth forms the core around which those ideas merge. Negative self-worth is the most important factor that nurses must change in themselves in order to communicate from a healing perspective. This chapter focuses on the general nature of effective communication in the helping process.

THERAPEUTIC COMMUNICATION

Certain identifiable elements characterize therapeutic or healing communication. In the nurse-client interaction, the nurse should be:

* **Fully present**—Totally focused on the client and his or her ideas about the situation. Does not get lost in memories of "clients past" or in his or her own present or future problems. Allows interaction with the client to command his or her full attention.
* **Listening**—Listens with the whole self in order to ascertain the client's meanings and goals. Clarifies interpretations of what is heard. Resists categorizing or projecting personal beliefs and values. Resists giving quick advice or telling the client what to do.
* **Speaking**—Communicates hope not just with an expression of ideas but with the ability to translate those ideas from an inner conviction

to an outer clarity. Self-awareness enables the speaker to voice articulately well-thought-out ideas regarding the role of the client in the healing process.
* **Developing trust**—Asks questions to ascertain the truth about the situation as the client perceives it. Communicates that the client is worth listening to, that he or she has important information to add to this process. Conveys the values of expertise and confidentiality, and never neglects the opportunity for informed consent so that the client feels that trust has been appropriately placed.

Thus, the therapeutic use of oneself includes communication that places the client in a position of informed equal, inevitably responsible for any positive outcomes in the helping process.

A CLOSER LOOK AT INTERPERSONAL INTERACTION

A key element of therapeutic communication is having an *attitude of respect* for the client. Respect includes a nonjudgmental approach and a belief that the client is capable of learning and growing. Ultimately, clients are entitled to manage their own lives in a way that is best for them. As obvious as this may seem, it is not always easy to have a nonjudgmental attitude. This attitude of acceptance can be quite challenging when one disapproves of the client's behaviors. Approving of the client's behavior is not the same as acceptance. It is not necessary to approve. It is possible to understand why the client has made certain life choices. For example, a client may be involved in an illegal activity and was raised in an environment where this activity was commonplace. It is still possible to respect the dignity and worth of this client as a person despite disagreeing with his or her lifestyle choices or behaviors. The nurse can practice being nonjudgmental by giving undivided attention when listening and by refraining from offering advice. Suspending judgment is facilitated by purposefully viewing the situation from the client's point of view.

There are several possible interpersonal processes within the nurse-client relationship that must be understood.

Sympathy involves having similar feelings about something. If the nurse is in agreement with the important that the nurse build a support system of friends and colleagues to meet those needs.

If the nurse crosses over a relationship boundary with the client, the interaction will confuse the client, and the nurse will appear to be offering more of him- or herself to the relationship than is facilitative to the helper-client relationship. In a therapeutic relationship, interaction will take place at levels five, four, and three with an occasional interchange at level two, but never at level one.

New professionals may confuse appropriate boundaries and find themselves making errors in judgment, such as spending more time with one client than others in their care because that client meets their needs in some way. The nurse may also avoid a client and neglect his or her needs because something about the relationship is disturbing or anxiety provoking. When the client feels compelled to put the nurse at ease or meet the nurse's needs, a boundary has been crossed. Clients do not need this added anxiety; they need to relax and trust that the nurse has the client's best interests at heart and can manage the healing interaction free of awkwardness or threats to confidentiality and trust.

BELIEFS OF EFFECTIVE HELPERS

A.W. Combs[7] and colleagues at the University of Florida conducted research on the characteristics of effective helpers and concluded:

Good helpers are not born, nor are they made in the sense of being taught... Becoming a helper is a time-consuming process. It is not simply a matter of learning methods or of acquiring gadgets and gimmicks. It is a deeply personal process of exploration and discovery, the growth of unique individuals learning over a period of time how to use themselves effectively for helping other people.

In their study, helpers were evaluated for their effectiveness, and the most effective responded to specific questions about their beliefs in six major categories. The results are summarized in Table 2-1.

Professionals will act according to what they believe to be their purpose. The purpose of a therapeutic relationship is to listen carefully so that you will come to know your client and understand his or her health needs from the client's perspective. With this understanding, the nurse can use the nursing process and collaborate with other members of the health care team to promote self-care and the highest level of functioning possible.

Carl Rogers[8] suggests seven key questions that lead to a form of self-examination that will help us evaluate the quality of one's helping skills.

1. Can I behave in some way that will be perceived by the other person as trustworthy, as dependable or consistent in some deep sense? Here congruence is the key factor. Whatever feeling or attitude is being experienced must be matched by an awareness of that attitude, and actions must match feelings.

2. Can I be expressive enough as a person that what I am will be communicated unambiguously? The difficulty here is to be fully aware of who one truly is. Rogers says this: "...If I can form a helping relationship to myself—if I can be sensitively aware of and acceptant toward my own feelings—then the likelihood is great that I can form a helping relationship toward another."

3. Can I let myself experience positive attitudes toward this other person—attitudes of warmth, caring, liking, interest, respect? This often engenders the fear that if we allow ourselves to openly express these feelings, the client might misinterpret our intentions, and the therapeutic distance might be blurred. The key here is to remain in our professional identities and yet still relate in a caring way to the other person.

4. Can I be strong enough as a person to be separate from the other? This question speaks to avoiding identification. I must be ever aware of my own feelings and express them as mine, totally separate from the feelings I may perceive that the client is experiencing. Likewise, I must be strong in my otherness to avoid becoming depressed when my client is depressed, or fearful in the face of my client's fear, or destroyed by his or her anger.

5. Can I let myself enter fully into the world of my client's feelings and personal meanings and see these as he or she does? The key effort here is to avoid judging the client's perspectives, but instead allow empathy to occur. In this way, once the world of the other is more fully experienced, the help that is offered can be based

---

Table 2-1

SUMMARY OF THE BELIEFS OF "EFFECTIVE" HELPERS

Combs and associates describe commonly held beliefs and perceptions of effective helpers in six categories:

1. Subject or Discipline

One is committed to knowing one's discipline well, and knowledge about one's discipline is so personally integrated and meaningful as to have the quality of beliefs. Effective helpers are committed to discovering the personal meaning of knowledge and converting it to beliefs.

2. Helper's Frame of Reference

Effective helpers tend to favor an internal frame of reference emphasizing the importance of people's attitudes, feelings, and values that are uniquely human over an external frame of reference that emphasizes facts, things, organization, money, etc.

3. Beliefs About People

Effective helpers believe that people are essentially:

* Able to understand and deal with their own problems given sufficient time and information
* Friendly and well-intentioned
* Worthy and have great value; they possess dignity and integrity that must be maintained
* Internally motivated, maturing from within and striving to grow and help themselves
* A source of satisfaction in professional work rather than a source of suspicion and frustration

4. Helper's Self-Concept

Effective helpers have a clear sense of self before they enter into relationships with others. They feel basically fulfilled and adequate, so self-discipline is well practiced. Therapeutic presence for the other is made possible by a strong sense of self, of personal fulfillment, and of personal adequacy.

5. Helper's Purposes

Effective helpers believe that their purpose is to facilitate and assist rather than control people. Their purpose includes honesty, acknowledging personal inadequacies, and need for growth. Another purpose is to be involved and committed to the helping process. They are committed to working out solutions rather than working toward preconceived goals or notions.

6. Beliefs About Appropriate Methods or Approaches to the Task

Effective helpers are more oriented toward people than toward rules and regulations. They are more concerned about people's perceptions than with the objective framework within which they practice. In helping people, the most effective approach is to discover how the world seems to that person. Self-concept is at the heart of the way one views the world, and so working with self-concept is imperative. Helpers have to be committed to gaining the trust of clients so that self-control can be relearned in a positive way. The helping relationship makes this growth possible.

Reprinted with permission from Combs AW. *Florida Studies in the Helping Professions*. Gainesville, Fla: University of Florida Press; 1969.

on this holistic level of knowing made possible by empathy. Meanings can be confronted with acceptance and modified to work toward healing. Judgment and criticism of meanings places a barrier between the helper and the client.

6. Can I act with sufficient sensitivity that my behavior will not be perceived as a threat in the relationship? A client who feels free of external fear or threat feels free to examine behavior and change it. Client care is threatening in and of itself. Whatever we can do to lower anxiety will assist the effectiveness of our helping.

7. Can I meet this other individual as a person who is in the process of becoming, or will I be bound by his or her past and by my past? Martin Buber[9] uses the phrase "confirming the other." This means accepting the whole potentiality of the other... the person he or she was created to become. People will act the way we relate to them. The Pygmalion effect was described following the famous Broadway play in which a poor working girl showed that she could behave like a princess when she was treated like one and taught carefully.

CONCLUSION

The more a nurse fully comprehends the importance of the nature of helping, the more the nurse will become committed to the growth required for consistent therapeutic use of self. Practice and study are necessary for improvement. Discussing confusing interactions with a mentor or experienced colleague can be very helpful in preventing errors in judgment or at least learning from experiences so that they will not be repeated.

REFERENCES

1. Peplau HE. *Interpersonal Relations in Nursing.* New York: Putnam; 1952.
2. Davis CM. What is empathy and can empathy be taught? *Physical Therapy.* 1990;70:707-715.
3. Breggin PR. *The Heart of Being Helpful.* New York; Springer; 1997.
4. Stein E. *On the Problem of Empathy.* 2nd ed. The Hague, Martinus Nijhoff; 1970.
5. Goleman D. *Emotional Intelligence.* New York: Bantam Books; 1995.
6. Powell J. *Why Am I Afraid to Tell You Who I Am?* Niles, Ill: Argus Communications; 1969.
7. Combs AW, Avila DL, Purkey WW. *Helping Relationships—Basic Concepts for the Health Professions.* 2nd ed. Boston: Allyn and Bacon, Inc; 1971.
8. Rogers C. The characteristics of a helping relationship. In Rogers C, ed. *On Becoming a Person.* Boston: Houghton Mifflin; 1961.
9. Buber M, Rogers C. Personal communication (transcription). April 18, 1957.

EXERCISES

1. What Is My Communication Style?

* What I like most about the way I communicate with others is...

* I am most comfortable communicating when...

* I am most uncomfortable communicating when...

* What I want to change about the way I communicate with others is...

* I don't know how to say...

* When I want to express my thoughts to loved ones, I usually...

* When I want to communicate my feelings to loved ones, I usually...

* When I have to communicate upsetting information, I usually...

Discussion

After you have answered these questions, write a summary of your communication style. In what ways will your communication style affect your relationships with colleagues? With clients?

2. Responding to Situations

Below are situations in which you might find yourself as you interact with clients in the clinical setting. These situations are posed to help you better understand the process of therapeutic interaction.

A. Your client, Mr. Jefferson, is 70 years old and has several health problems including obesity, diabetes, and hypertension. When you visit him in his home to conduct health teaching, you notice that he doesn't seem interested in what you have to say. When you ask about how he has been managing his diabetes, he changes the subject.

* What might you feel in this situation?

* What questions could you ask to find out what health issues are important to him?

* What conflicts might exist between his needs and yours?

B. Mrs. Weslan, age 45, has a long history of severe psychiatric problems and has a diagnosis of bipolar disorder. She is hospitalized briefly for stabilization with medications, and you are assigned to develop a therapeutic relationship with her. Her problems seem overwhelming and you wonder where to begin.

* What might you be feeling in this situation?

* Is there really anything that you can do that will help?

* What would be a rewarding outcome in this situation?

* What might be one realistic therapeutic goal in this situation?

Discussion

In your self-assessment notebook, summarize what you have learned about yourself in doing these exercises. What kinds of clients might you be interested in working with when you graduate? What factors have influenced your preferences?

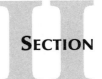

Interacting With Others

The Process of Helping

Christine L. Williams, DNSc, RN, BC and Carol M. Davis, PT, EdD, MS, FAPTA

OBJECTIVES

1. To describe the characteristics of a helping interview
2. To portray the qualities of an effective interviewer
3. To emphasize the importance of both thoughts and feelings in communication
4. To emphasize the importance of effective communication in the initial stages of the relationship

Therapeutic interaction requires new skills, but more than that, it requires unlearning old ways of communicating that will not work in a therapeutic relationship. This chapter is devoted to teaching a new way of communicating with the express purpose of developing therapeutic presence with clients.

Remember that the client is not simply the person with an illness or injury, but his or her entire family is your "client" as well. Be aware of the need to include family members in your assessment and planning. Even when the "identified client" wants your help, the cooperation of supportive family members can make the difference between success and failure of the plan of care.

When clients are ill, they often feel afraid and vulnerable. They may be in the midst of a major life crisis such as birth or death. They may be caring for a family member who is dying. Most people resist giving over some control of their lives to strangers. They may not welcome this encounter with a nurse. The underlying theme in this chapter is to help you communicate in ways that foster opportunities for growth or solve problems while respecting and honoring clients during their health care experience.

As nurses, we recognize that the client may feel at a distinct disadvantage. At least from their perspective, we possess the knowledge and skills to manage the situation. Our interest, genuineness, acceptance, and positive regard are critical to establishing a healing relationship. The trust we foster will influence how much information we obtain during the assessment and how much the client benefits from our help.

THE HEALTH CARE ENCOUNTER

Without effective communication, we are unable to acquire objective and subjective information in order to make health care decisions with our clients, and we are unable to utilize the relationship between nurse and client for therapeutic ends. This chapter focuses on sorting out emotion-laden communication in order to help clients identify and solve their own problems. Sometimes the first encounter with a client is in the home or outpatient clinic. If there is no emergency, the nurse can focus on collecting broad to better understand the client. In other ncounters are brief, such as a bedside encounter in the hospital at 3:00 am when the nurse is monitoring the client's condition. The context of each interaction will affect the nature of the nurse's approach; however, many principles remain constant.

THE HEALTH CARE INTERVIEW: A UNIQUE FORM OF COMMUNICATING

The interview is the very first opportunity to convey a professional healing attitude, and it must be learned and practiced in order to develop skill. Learning therapeutic communication is like learning a new language. At first it will feel awkward. You will wonder if your words sound artificial. Gradually, as you practice, it will sound more and more natural. When you see the results in the trust and confidence of your clients, you will be encouraged to keep working at it.

Your words and inner attitude must be in harmony in order for the interview to be therapeutic. For the best results, the nurse must feel confident, peaceful, at one with his or her self, and genuinely willing to establish a healing relationship. Take a few deep breaths to relax before you begin. Focusing on the client's needs rather than your own feelings of awkwardness will help you to forget your self-consciousness.

Meeting the Client

Your introduction will include the use of your full name and the client's formal name. After the initial introduction, it is appropriate to ask the client what name he or she would like you to use. Many of us have had the experience of having our names mispronounced or shortened in ways that left us feeling vaguely and unnecessarily uncomfortable. Endearments such as "sweetie" or "mamma" are never appropriate. Your nonverbal behavior must convey respect and warmth. Position yourself at "eye" level rather than standing over the client as he or she lies in bed or sits in a wheelchair. Lean slightly toward the client to convey interest. Maintaining eye contact while staying at an appropriate social distance (4 feet away) is important in beginning a successful relationship.

Active Listening

Active listening is a form of therapeutic listening that helps the client clearly convey what he or she is trying to say. It involves paraphrasing the client's words in order to clarify whether or not you have caught the intended meaning. You must suspend your thoughts and attend exclusively to the words of the other person. **This is not easy** and requires practice. Your goal is to understand rather than judge or defend against. For some, it will require great effort to resist responding with a suggestion of what to do or with an argument. One word you will want to avoid at such times is "but..."

Active listening is made up of three different processes[1]:

1. **Restatement**—Repeating the words of the client as you have heard them.

   Example: "You better call the doctor because I'm leaving this hospital today!"

   Restatement: "You want the doctor to discharge you today?"

   Restatement can be annoying if not timed appropriately. When done well, it assures the client that you have, indeed, heard what he or she is saying. The main purpose of restatement is to help the client continue speaking and should only be used in the *initial phases* of active listening. Once you have reassured the client that you are hearing his or her words, reflection and clarification become more useful responses.

2. **Reflection**—Verbalizing both the content and the implied feelings of the speaker.

   Example: "No one seems to know what's wrong with me. I've had so many tests and no one tells me anything. I've had it!"

   Reflection: "You're tired of all the tests and frustrated because you still don't know what's wrong?"

   The purpose of reflection is to express in words the feelings and attitudes sensed behind the words of the speaker. This aspect of listening indicates you are hearing more than just the words—you are hearing the emotion behind them. Sometimes we guess incorrectly, but this gives the client the chance to clarify for us and for him- or herself exactly what he or she is feeling. Awareness of feelings is critical to identifying the real problem. When the nurse wants to help the client to examine both thoughts and feelings, clarification is used.

3. **Clarification**—Summarizing or simplifying the client's thoughts and feelings and resolving confused verbalizations into clear, concise statements.

   Example: "When the doctor told me I needed some tests, I thought I would be out of here in a couple of days. But I've been sitting here all weekend doing nothing and now you're telling me I still need more tests. I can't stay here; I need to get back to work. I'm not sure what I'm supposed to do. I can't afford to just lie around here another day."

   Clarification: "When you came into the hospital on Thursday you thought you would be discharged by the weekend? Now you realize that the tests are going to take longer than you expected and you are worried about missing work?"

   These skills take practice, as does resisting the answer that tends toward "fixing" the problem. In this case, the client may begin to feel some relief just because he or she has been heard and may begin to problem solve on his or her own: "I will call my supervisor and explain that I haven't had a chance to talk to the doctor yet. I don't really want to leave if there is something really wrong."

Nonverbal Communication

We communicate more with nonverbal behavior than we do with words. Our nonverbal behavior conveys how we feel regardless of what we say. The nurse's nonverbal communication can either facilitate or hinder the quality of the interview. Key nonverbal elements of a helping interview include use of space (eliminate physical barriers such as a desk between you and the client), time (minimize interruptions), appropriate posture (avoiding rigid posture, slouching, or defiant gestures), voice inflection (appropriate speed and volume; warmth and genuine interest conveyed vs flatness or excessive use of "you knows"), and eliminating distracting body movements (twitching, shaking foot, tapping pencil).

Congruence

Congruence is a term that indicates that the verbal and nonverbal messages match.[2] For example, congruence is present when the nurse admits that he or she is frustrated or irritated rather than denying those feelings. If the nurse denies feelings, nonverbal responses such as muscle tension and facial expression will communicate the feeling the the client anyway and create confusion. Incongruence is present when the nurse denies anger but says it with clenched fists. Incongruence appears dishonest or "not ringing true." How often have we been caught in incongruence when someone asks for a compliment: "Well, do you like my new haircut or *not*?" "Well, yes, it's okay, I guess." What was felt was less than okay but no one likes to appear rude. When a person is congruent, he or she appears open, honest, genuine, and authentic. Nonverbal cues and tone of voice are consistent with the words spoken.

Congruence requires self-awareness. Before speaking, you must consider both feelings and thoughts and reconcile conflicts such as wanting not to be hurtful, yet wanting to be honest. A congruent response to the requested compliment might be: "You know, I noticed you had a new haircut, but I really liked it the old way." With this response, the person realizes that you value honesty and are willing to be honest, but can avoid being rude. The message "rings true" and you feel better. More important, the person knows you will resist trying to please others and disregarding your own feelings.

Congruence is best conveyed when it is communicated with sensitivity. It should never be used as a rationalization for insensitive and rude "honesty."

Communicating Emotions

Many of us are rather unaware of our day-to-day communication style and are surprised when someone misunderstands the message we have tried to convey. It is difficult to come outside of ourselves and watch ourselves interact with others, and to reflect on our feelings and the way in which we react to others. Some of us have been given direct feedback about our communication. Statements such as "I love the way you listen carefully to what I say and wait until I'm finished before you respond" vs "I wish you'd hear me out instead of mentally practicing a quick comeback!" give us clear information about how we are doing as we communicate in that moment.

When strong emotions are communicated, the message may be unclear because the client (or nurse) is upset and unable to clearly identify what the heart of the problem is and how to best go about solving it. As a nurse, you must be aware of your emotional reactions and avoid using emotion-laden communication (even when you feel personally attacked) in order to maximize your therapeutic effectiveness.

Emotion-laden exchanges are cluttered with intense feelings, derogatory remarks, apologies, etc. In order to sort out the problem, special listening skills are needed to defuse the emotion and get at the problem. Critical to this method is resisting the desire to respond (unhelpfully) in a way to "fix" it quickly in order to get rid of the anger or conflict. The alternative is to listen and resist the quick advice or defensive reply.

Case Example

Mrs. Mendel, an 82-year-old widow, is admitted to a nursing home accompanied by her daughter Mrs. Garcia. Mrs. Mendel has lived with her daughter for the past 10 years however, in the past year she has become increasingly confused and disoriented, and her resistance to eating, bathing, and dressing has made it difficult for her daughter to manage. Her illness is diagnosed as dementia. Mrs. Garcia made the reluctant decision to place her mother in a nursing home and was feeling tremendous guilt about it. She had promised her mother that she would always care for her at home.

Mrs. Garcia visited every day and was often present during mealtimes. Although Mrs. Mendel was gaining weight, Mrs. Garcia was critical of her mother's care and especially the quality of the meals. One day she came to the nurses' station and shouted, "The food you are giving my mother is completely unacceptable. You can't expect her to eat that!"

This is an example of an emotion-laden interaction similar to many that take place daily in hospitals and long-term care facilities. If you were the nurse, how would you have responded? What would you have felt? Would you have become defensive? Would you have argued that Mrs. Mendel was showing remarkable signs of improvement now that she was at the nursing home? Would you have shouted, "Nobody speaks to me like that!"?

Situations such as placing a loved one in long-term care involve feelings of loss, vulnerability, and fear. Family members must give over control to strangers, often in institutions that seem strange, impersonal, and frightening with cultures very different from their own. At the root of every emotional outburst is a problem. What, exactly, is the problem in this case example, and whose problem is it? Mrs. Garcia would say that the problem is that her mother is not being treated well. Therefore, the nursing home and food are the problems. The nurse might say that the problem is that Mrs. Garcia is feeling helpless about her mother's illness and lashed out in frustration. Both are correct from their own way of seeing the world. If the nurse maintains that he or she is "right," it will not solve the problem. In order to resolve the problem, it is the nurse's responsibility to take the client's view (in this case, Mrs. Garcia, as Mrs. Mendel's closest relative is the client). The nurse can resolve this uncomfortable situation and at the same time avoid taking blame for the situation by the use of "I" messages.

Clear Sending— Use of "I" Statements

When an individual feels distressed and wants to communicate to another person that he or she is upset, clear communication is facilitated with "I" messages ("I think" or "I feel"); rather than the commonly used editorial "they," "you," or "everyone" are most effective for resolving problems. Many people have a tendency to blame when they feel uncomfortable. An example in which the nurse blames the client might be: "You keep making suggestive remarks. I'm not going to be able to help you if you keep talking that way." In this case, whose problem is it? If I am upset the problem is mine. The following response using an "I" message is more likely to resolve the problem: "I'm feeling very frustrated. I'm trying to help you learn about your diabetes and I'm feeling uncomfortable with the things you are saying. Let's talk about this."

With "I" messages, the nurse clearly expresses and takes responsibility for his or her frustration. This way, it is up to the other person to respond, hopefully with concern, perhaps even with active listening. Note, however, that use of an "I" statement does not guarantee that the other person will respond in a helpful way. What it does mean is that the nurse's feelings will be expressed appropriately and those feelings will be less likely to disrupt the relationship. If those feelings are not expressed, they may lead to the nurse avoiding this client, who is in need of diabetic teaching.

Using "I" statements involves taking a risk. When the nurse speaks in the first person, he or she takes responsibility for feelings rather than ignoring, disclaiming, or minimizing them. It takes reflective thought to decide what the nurse is feeling and how it can be expressed appropriately. Sending "I" messages tells the other person that you believe this problem can be solved with appropriate, clear, respectful discussion.

The nurse can let Mrs. Garcia know that she is a valued member of the health care team and that her contributions to her mother's care are essential to her well-being. A response that helps to establish the nurse's desire to work together with Mrs. Garcia might be "I see that you are very upset and I want to help. Let's sit and talk about this. Please tell me what is wrong." With this approach, the nurse may learn that it is not the food at all that is the problem but that Mrs. Garcia is feeling overwhelmed by many events in her life. After allowing her to express her frustration, Mrs. Garcia and the nurse may decide that bringing in food from home is one small step toward helping her feel less helpless and to be more involved in her mother's care. When the nurse communicates in a helpful manner, he or she resists the need to respond impulsively, to offer quick advice, or to offer a quick solution to a problem. Instead, the nurse strives to clarify the problem and to assist the person in solving it for him- or herself.

Unhelpful Responses

Unhelpful responses are impulsive and do not reflect caring, warmth, respect, compassion, and empathy. Accepting that the other person is doing the best he or she can in the moment and accepting the responsibility to be therapeutic in the midst of a chaotic situation are actions of a mature health professional.

* **Offering false reassurances.** Statements such as "She'll be fine, she just needs time to adjust" signal the nurse's unwillingness to listen to clients' perceptions of their problems.
* **Dismissing concerns.** Statements such as "Oh, it can't be all that bad" or "If you think you have

it bad, you should just look around you" may be used by a nurse who is trying to get away as rapidly as possible.
* **Offering judgmental responses.** There are several types of judgmental responses, such as responses that convey approval or disapproval, either verbally or nonverbally, at an inappropriate moment. One such verbal response is, "You're really planning to take the baby home to a hotel room?" Another response gives advice at a time when it is more important for the client to make his or her own decision, such as, "You need to leave your husband now before things get any worse!" Another response that is stereotypical and not helpful is "All parents have to make sacrifices."
* **Defensiveness.** When we feel threatened, we respond defensively. Defensiveness indicates a personalization and refusal to listen carefully to what the client is saying. A response such as "We are so understaffed. I am trying to take care of your mother's needs but I have eight other residents to take care of" may be true, but does little to solve the daughter's problem.

As you practice viewing the world from the client's perspective you will more than likely receive cooperation from clients. This view places you in the role of advocate and partner rather than that of authority figure or adversary.

The Helping Interview

Interviewing is much more than obtaining a client's history. The interview often sets the stage for the care we give. A client may be seeking health information or may be worried or in pain. He or she may feel in need of our help and understanding. Clients hope that we will listen carefully and that we will know something about their concerns.

Helpful Attitudes

Not only is it important to convey an accepting attitude for our clients during the interview, it is imperative that the client feels listened to and understood so that all of the important information can surface that will lead to the most adequate and complete understanding of the client's concern. Thus, effective clinical decision-making depends on skillful interviewing.

The Healing Attitude of the Interview

Clients are simply people who need our professional help to identify their health needs and to help them to achieve their best possible health state. Nurses who have an attitude that facilitates healing are able to accept their clients just as they are, without judging them. These nurses will have identified and dealt with their own biases and prejudices about certain behaviors such as alcohol abuse, smoking, use of profanity, lack of motivation to change, obesity, etc. They will have determined that they are willing to be therapeutic even when the client does not behave as the nurse would. As much as possible, they will be aware of and willing to put aside prejudices about culture and ethnicity, gender, age, or sexual orientation. As much as we might dislike a client's behavior, it is helpful to believe that the client would have acted differently if he or she had more information and had been less impulsive.

The key information that is obtained in the interview includes the following:

* What is the reason for this health care encounter?
* What is the client's perception of the problem?
* What does the client expect from this interaction? What does he or she hope that you will do?
* What is the exact nature of the health care concern?
* What are the characteristics of the situation? When did it begin? Precipitating factors? What alleviates the problem? What makes it worse? What factors are associated with it?

More on the Interview Attitude: What We Are

Alfred Benjamin[4] says:

When interviewing, we are left with what we are. We have no books then, no classroom lessons, and no supporting person at our elbow. We are alone with the individual who has come to seek our help. How can we assist him (or her)? The same basic issues will confront us afresh whenever we face an interviewee for the first time. In summary they are:

* Shall we allow ourselves to emerge as genuine human beings, or shall we hide behind our role, position, and authority?

* Shall we really try to listen with all our senses to the interviewee?
* Shall we try to understand him (her) with empathy and acceptance?
* Shall we interpret his (her) behavior to him (her) in terms of his (her) frame of reference, our own, or society's?
* Shall we evaluate his (her) thoughts, feelings, and actions, and if so, in terms of whose values: his (hers), society's, or ours?
* Shall we support, encourage, urge him (her) on so that by leaning on us hopefully he (she) may be able to rely on his (her) own strength one day?
* Shall we question and probe, push and prod, causing him (her) to feel that we are in command and that once all our queries have been answered, we shall provide the solutions he (she) is seeking?
* Shall we guide him (her) in the direction we feel certain is the best for him (her)?
* Shall we reject his (her)... thoughts and feelings, and insist that he (she) become like us, or at least conform to our perception of what he (she) should become?

The Interview

Timing

With regard to timing, an effective interviewer avoids interrupting (which often reveals an underlying harmful attitude of "this person is not very important to me") and listens carefully using silence. Nurses who are uncomfortable with silence will miss much of what a person says if the client were given a chance to pause and reflect. A specific amount of time is set to spend listening to the client as he or she tells you his or her story. The amount of time will vary with the situation. Generally, less time is available in an emergency and more time is allotted when the client's need is for health promotion.

The most accurate accounting of the reason for seeking help is gained through listening to the client's "story." This information does not always follow the structured format that is found on a data collection form, but by allowing the client to explain the situation in his or her own way, most important information will come up. The nurse can fill in the gaps later. If the client is highly anxious, he or she will need the nurse's guidance to explain fully. Guidance should be kept to a minimum to determine what the client believes is important and what he or she is seeking in this encounter. General information is obtained first, allowing the client to become comfortable and to begin in his or her own way. More specific requests for information, especially sensitive information, can be obtained later, once rapport has developed.

Stages of the Interview

There are four stages in the interview: the preparation phase, orientation phase, working phase, and termination phase.

Probably the most difficult part of communicating with clients is getting started. Students often delay meeting their clients to read health records or obtain information from other nurses. Although these activities have value, there is no substitute for communicating directly with the client. Anticipation of the encounter can lead to a number of concerns, such as will the client like me? Will he or she refuse to talk to me? What should I do if the client's family is visiting or if the client is talking on the phone?

The *preparation phase* takes place before meeting the client. Clinical supervision is an important part of the preparation process and is used as an ongoing method of helping to improve therapeutic communication skills. It is critical to meet with a faculty member or, for the practicing nurse, an experienced clinician to discuss any concerns about meeting with the client and how to proceed. Guidance from a more experienced person is considered an integral part of professional practice. Through the relationship with a supervisor, the student or nurse learns more about the therapeutic use of self. The supervisor can assist the nurse in examining his or her feelings about the client.

To assist in the process of supervision, the interview may be audiotaped or videotaped. This allows an accurate review and critique of the interaction. When taping is impossible due to institutional policies, process recording can be substituted. In process recording, the student or nurse writes the conversation verbatim from memory immediately following the interview. The written version is shared with the supervisor and discussed. Although this process is not as accurate as recording an interview as it happens, it is a useful learning tool.

Kotecki[3] identified a process called *affirming the self* that was used by student nurses to prepare for communicating with clients. Affirming the self consists of using techniques such as positive self-talk to improve their readiness to engage in a new relationship with clients. Each of us engages in an inner dialogue continuously as we go about our daily activities. This dialogue can be self-critical, leading to increased anxiety and discomfort. For example, when students report self-talk, such as "This patient will be hard to talk to" or "I know I am going to make a fool of myself," their likely response will be anxiety. Under these circumstances, no wonder the student avoids the encounter! When self-talk is positive and supportive, students approach a new situation with confidence.for example, "I know I can handle this situation. I've been successful before, I can do it again." When we find ourselves engaging in negative self-talk, we can tell ourselves to "Stop!" and redirect our thoughts to a more positive theme.

Consider the environment you have chosen for the interview to be sure it is as comfortable as possible. Temperature, lighting, and seating arrangements are examples of factors that can influence how much the client is willing to talk. In the hospital or home, the nurse needs to have comfortable seating as well as the client. If the nurse is standing, this sends a message "I am not staying long." The client's inner state is important as well. The client is not likely to communicate freely if he or she is in pain or suffers other physical discomforts. Take the time to provide comfort first.

Your demeanor will also influence the client's reaction to the encounter. Is your manner of dress that of a competent professional? Your self-esteem is reflected in the care you take with your appearance. Your style of dress communicates messages about how you view your role as a nurse. The client will be more likely to develop trust in an individual who is self-assured and professional in appearance. Identification badges are important as well. When the client can read your name and title, he or she can be assured of who you are and what he or she can expect.

The *orientation phase* of the interview takes place as you, the interviewer, meet the client and explain who you are, why you are here, the purpose of the interview, and the amount of time you will spend with the client. Termination of the relationship begins at this initial step as you clarify what to expect. Be as clear as you can about how long this interview will last and whether future sessions are anticipated. It is important to provide as much privacy as possible at the first meeting so that the client will be comfortable about bringing up his or her concerns. Although you may feel rushed, communicate patience and attentiveness in order to be effective. On a busy morning, you may have only 5 minutes to spend with a client, but you can give the client your undivided attention for those 5 minutes and arrange to come back later to continue the interview.

Establishing rapport is facilitated by beginning with a brief social exchange. This type of communication is called the "ice breaker." It is a way of making the client comfortable before the business of the interview begins. Whether you are visiting a client in a health care setting or in his or her home, you can use the environment to get clues about how to begin. Asking about a greeting card or family photographs displayed on a bedside table are examples of ice breakers. The client may have been engaged in an activity, such as a hobby, just before you arrived. By asking about the activity, you show your interest in the client as a person rather than simply a health care "problem."

The body of the interview is the *working phase*. In this stage, rapport has been developed and the client begins to discuss his or her health issues. A good interviewer will guide the client, assisting the client to explore his or her situation, but not allowing the conversation to drift from the focus of the interaction. Active listening helps the client to clarify the unique aspects of his or her story. The interviewer listens carefully and sorts the information, jotting down significant revelations as he or she prepares for the clinical examination. The body of the interview unfolds in a unique story that the client is encouraged to tell. The helpful interviewer communicates to the client that he or she is being heard by a skilled and caring nurse. When moving from one topic to another, it is helpful to use a transition statement. An example would be: "I think I understand about your headaches; I'd like to hear about your sleep patterns now."

The *termination phase* of the interview takes place at a time that has been predetermined by the interviewer. If it becomes obvious that the interview is not complete, the interviewer does not just let the session drop but says, for example, "We're beginning to run out of time for this session and I realize you haven't yet finished. What needs to be covered still?" Then a second session is scheduled. It is advisable to complete the discussion of the problem before beginning the physical examination. As an interviewer you will be dividing your attention if you try to obtain meaningful

information while engaging in palpation and physical evaluation methods. Further, the client will feel vulnerable and exposed, and is less likely to share information.

In an ongoing relationship with a client, there may be several meetings over a period of time. When the time of termination is known, it is the nurse's responsibility to give adequate preparation so that termination does not come as a surprise. The client already knows approximately when the relationship will end because you provided the information during the orientation phase. Reminders about termination should come at the beginning of any session rather than at the end in order to give the client adequate opportunity to discuss it. The client needs an opportunity to discuss what has been gained and to express any unmet needs. The nurse can then make referrals for additional health care if needed.

Sometimes clients resist ending an interview. Establishing trust involves telling the client what to expect and following through on what you have promised. If a home visit is scheduled to be 1 hour, for example, it is best to leave as scheduled rather than be persuaded to stay longer without any clear purpose. If important concerns prolong the meeting, discuss the change and renegotiate the time frame for the visit. Sometimes the client seems to be prolonging the session unnecessarily. In this case, congruence is conveyed by stating that you are leaving and then walking in the direction of the door, as opposed to stating that you are leaving but remaining seated as the client continues to talk.

These are the central attitudinal questions that underlie every helping interview. When you read the above questions carefully, you will see that Benjamin phrases a few to encourage a negative response, as if to have us examine our attitudes very carefully in order to be clear about our helping intentions. Once a healing attitude is established, skillful and artful questions will follow, and the interview will become one more important tool in the nurse's repertoire of healing behaviors. When this routine becomes second nature, less stress will be attached to it and you will experience great pleasure listening to most of your clients tell their story.

CONCLUSION

If you have ever been fortunate enough to have observed an experienced nurse at work, you have seen a person who truly values the interview and devotes the kind of attention to it described in this chapter. The greatest obstacles to consistent use of the helping interview are overwork and burnout. The more we feel overextended in our day and the more we feel that we are repeatedly facing irresolvable problems, the more difficult it will be to come outside of ourselves with a therapeutic presence during the interview. The very foundation of the helping interview is a commitment to keeping a balance in our lives so that we are rested and have the energy to give to our work. We have a right to keep a reasonable pace. It is our responsibility to make sure we have as much of ourselves to give as we can.

REFERENCES

1. Munson PJ, Johnson RB. *Humanizing Instruction or Helping Your Students Up the Staircase*. Chapel Hill, NC: Johnson Self Instructional Package; 1972.

2. Rogers CR. *The Therapeutic Relationship and Its Impact*. Madison, Wis: University of Wisconsin Press; 1967.

3. Kotecki CN. Baccalaureate nursing students' communication process in the clinical setting. *J Nurs Educ*. 2002;41(2):61-68.

4. Benjamin A. *The Helping Interview*. 2nd ed. Boston: Houghton Mifflin; 1969.

EXERCISES

1. Becoming a Professional Helper

In your self-assessment notebook, respond to each of the following questions:

✳ I first became aware that I wanted to help others when…

✳ I feel good when I know I have helped another because…

✳ I prefer helping people who…

✳ When someone refuses my help, I feel…

✳ When someone does not seem to help him- or herself, I feel…

Discussion

After answering each of the above questions, summarize the major reasons that you decided to make helping others your life's work. What is rewarding about helping others? What frustrations may occur in helping others? How will you achieve a balance between helping and encouraging self-reliance?

2. Responding to Situations

Following are situations in which you might find yourself as you interact with clients in the clinical setting. These situations are posed to help you explore what you might feel and say in the situation.

A. You are scheduled to interview Mr. Reynolds in his home and report your findings to your clinical instructor. There has been a misunderstanding about the time of your visit, and Mr. Reynolds has been waiting for you for over an hour, pacing up and down. When you go to introduce yourself to him, he turns to you angrily and says, "You don't give a damn about other people's time. Don't you realize how long I've been waiting?"

✳ How might you feel at this moment?

✳ What feelings do you think the client is experiencing?

✳ What are some specific things you might say or do at this point to try to demonstrate empathy?

B. You walk into a client's room, and he is watching television. You introduce yourself, and the patient never even takes his eyes off the TV. He acts as if you are not present in the room.

  ✶ How might you feel?

  ✶ What might be the client's situation?

  ✶ What self-talk strategies might you use to manage your discomfort in this situation?

C. You are completing an initial assessment on a child who has been admitted to the hospital. The child and her mother are homeless, and the child has an acute upper respiratory infection. The child's clothes are old and dirty, and it appears that she has not been bathed in a long time.

  ✶ What might you feel?

  ✶ What approaches to communicating would be helpful? Not helpful?

D. You are trying to conduct an interview with an 85-year-old client, but each time you ask her a question, her adult daughter answers it for her.

  ✶ What might you feel?

  ✶ What might be underlying this situation?

  ✶ What are some things you might say or do to get more information from the client herself?

E. You are interviewing a client and he suddenly leans forward, grabs your arm, and says, "You are so attractive. Are you married?"

  ✶ How might you feel?

  ✶ What might be underlying the client's behavior?

  ✶ What might you say or do to get the interview back on track?

Discussion

In your self-assessment notebook, summarize what you have learned about yourself in completing these exercises. Which of the above situations would be most challenging for you? Are there other situations that you can think of that might be uncomfortable for you? Write about a client situation different from those listed above that would be awkward or uncomfortable. Write about what you would feel and how you might respond appropriately.

3. Active Listening

Active listening involves restatement (of the words of the sender), reflection (of the words and underlying feelings of the sender), and clarification (summarizes and focuses the sender's message). Practice writing all three types of responses as requested below.

RESTATEMENT

Client	*Response from You*
"I'm very worried about my husband's blood sugar. It seems to be very high most days."	"You're worried about your husband's blood sugar being so high."
"I used to be able to walk up a flight of stairs without stopping, but now I can only climb one or two steps."	
"The nurse practitioner told me about several treatment options to consider. I just don't know what to do."	

REFLECTION

Client	*Response from You*
"This pain has been going on for months now. I just wish someone would fix it for me."	"Your pain just drags on and you wish to relieve it. Perhaps you're concerned that it will never go away?"
"Yesterday was a good day, but today I feel the same old way."	
"It's hard remembering to do my exercises. I want to get better, but it's hard."	

CLARIFICATION

Client

"I wish someone would tell me what's going on with my knees. When I get up in the morning they're fine, but by noon they're swollen and feel tired. I'm too young to be suffering with joint problems. Is this arthritis or what? Do I have to live with this forever?"

Response from You

"You're worried that your knee problem might be arthritis and that you'll never be rid of it?"

"When they told me my son had learning problems I just didn't know what to think. I don't believe in giving a child mind-altering pills, but his teachers say he is failing at school. I don't know how to help him."

"I almost didn't make it here. I got a horrible headache as I was driving here. The traffic is so stressful in this city. Will it ever end? New cars every day on the road. I don't know if I can keep up driving with these headaches. Is there anything you can do for me?"

Communication Strategies

Christine L. Williams, DNSc, RN, BC

OBJECTIVES

1. To compare different types of questions used in communicating with clients and to use in various situations
2. To list different types of questions and situations appropriate to their use
3. To describe a progression of questioning
4. To discuss therapeutic communication strategies
5. To analyze barriers to therapeutic communication
6. To delineate guidelines for conveying upsetting information

LEARNING NEW COMMUNICATION SKILLS

Fear of not knowing what to say is a common concern voiced by many students[1] and nurses alike. Nurses sometimes worry that they will not know what to say or will say the wrong thing. This is a normal part of being uncomfortable in an unfamiliar situation. These worries arise when the nurse is focusing on him- or herself rather than the client. These fears will lessen when the nurse focuses on what the client is experiencing in the situation. When the nurse is using empathy, it is more difficult to be self-conscious and awkward.

The art and science of nursing depends upon the skillful communication. The experienced nurse brings together a healthy sense of self, empathy and compassion, knowledge of the interview format, and constructive strategies for obtaining and conveying information. Everything we do or say communicates some kind of message. Therefore, it is important to master specific strategies that will facilitate the therapeutic relationship. In this chapter, guidelines for communicating in ways that are helpful will be presented.

QUESTIONING

Sometimes clients talk continuously with very few questions from the nurse. At other times, the client is very reluctant to share information and questioning becomes important in obtaining information. When the information the client offers is not sufficient for understanding health needs, skillful questioning can be used to obtain the missing information. There are many kinds of questions that can be used to obtain information, and some are more useful in therapeutic interactions.

Some questions are more threatening than others and must be reserved until rapport has developed. Asking about a client's feelings too early in the interaction can be perceived as threatening. This kind of questioning may result in the client becoming defensive or denying emotions. It can be difficult to face emotions and admit them to another person. Therefore, it is best to wait until the client has developed a degree of comfort in talking with you about his or her situation before you ask him or her to share feelings.

Progression of Questions

When meeting the client for the first time, the nurse guides the client to tell his or her complete "story." This includes an explanation of what has been happening in the client's life and what has happened that led to this encounter with the nurse. Certain types of questions are useful in getting the conversation started, while others are more helpful after rapport has developed.

The health care encounter begins with *broad openings*, such as "Tell me about yourself" or "Tell me about your family." Broad openings are designed to give the client the freedom to tell his or her story in whatever way is most comfortable. Often, clients skip over details that are important to the nurse; therefore, it is important to ask questions that will facilitate descriptions of events over time.

Describing

The *descriptive* question is used next to obtain information about what led to the health care encounter. Descriptive questions include those that begin with "Who?" "What?" "Where?" and "When?" When the reason for the health care encounter is illness or an accident, it is important to find out how it all began. Ask what happened or when the symptoms began. Descriptive questions can help the nurse to obtain a visual picture of the circumstances of an event, such as a seizure. Ask the client to describe where and when the event took place, who was there, what was said, and to place events in time sequence. This critical information should be documented with key statements quoted directly. It is the professional nurse's responsibility to conduct an initial assessment when a client is admitted to the health care system. Such specific information is useful for other members of the health care team and can prevent their asking the same sensitive questions over and over.

Open- and Closed-Ended Questions

Questions that are *open-ended* are worded to encourage the client to give explanations or to elaborate on a topic. These questions cannot be answered with one or two words. "What happened yesterday?" is an example of an open-ended question. Whenever possible, begin the conversation with open-ended questions. Open-ended questions are also useful later in the interaction to help the client express his or her feelings. "What is it like for you taking care of a sick child for so long?" Open-ended questions are extremely valuable in developing a therapeutic relationship. They provide direction and keep the conversation focused on health care concerns while allowing clients the opportunity to express their concerns in their own words. If the student practices asking open-ended questions when meeting a new client, he or she will often be surprised at how quickly rapport develops.

Closed-ended questions are worded in such a way that they can be answered in one or two words. Many times the nurse needs a specific piece of information and the closed-ended question is the most efficient way to obtain that information. For example, eventually in every admission interview the nurse asks, "Are you allergic to any medications?" Other examples of closed-ended questions include "What is today's date?" or "Are you in pain?" Although closed-ended questions are necessary at times, they can prevent the development of a smooth flow of conversation. It is best to avoid them at the beginning of a conversation unless a specific piece of information is needed urgently, such as "Did you take any insulin today?"

When nurses or student nurses are anxious, they are more likely to ask the client closed-ended questions one after another. This limits the flow of conversation to short answers and may lead to inferring that the client does not want to talk. If this happens, reflect on the format of your questions and switch to asking open-ended questions.

From General to Specific Questions

In some cases, clients have difficulty answering questions. The nurse may be interested in obtaining descriptions of the client's pain experience and begins the assessment with an open-ended question. "Tell me about your pain" may lead to no response or a limited response, such as "I don't know." It is always best to obtain information in the client's own words, but if the client is unable to explain, it may be necessary to provide some guidance. In these situations, the nurse progresses to more specific questions, such as a closed-ended question: "Does it hurt when I press here?" Another type of question that limits the client's response is the *forced-choice* question. The client must choose between two alternatives. Examples include "Is your pain sharp or dull?" and "Do you feel it more here or there?" Although useful, these questions do not encourage the client to answer with a more accurate alternative. Finally, the *laundry-list* question provides a series of choices: "Do you feel annoyed, frustrated, or angry?" These questions are less valuable because the client must choose from the list provided rather than putting the feeling into his or her own words. In some situations, such as clients with limited ability to speak, these questions may be effective in obtaining some response when the open-ended question leads only to silence.

Sharing Thoughts

Once the basic facts are obtained, the nurse encourages the client to describe his or her thoughts about the information. Each client has his or her own unique way of interpreting events, and these evaluations will influence the client's response to the events. With information about the client's thoughts, the nurse will uncover misinterpretations and misinformation that can be addressed in health teaching at a later time. For example, Mrs. Bouchard describes extreme conflict with her adolescent daughter over breaking a curfew. The nurse asks, "What did you think when your daughter did not come home on time?" Mrs. Bouchard replies that her daughter must not care about her parents very much because if she did she would not cause them to worry. The mother's conclusions about the meaning of her daughter's behavior caused an emotional response of hurt and anger that was not helpful to resolving the problem. The nurse also notes that the client will need teaching about adolescence and the issues related to that stage of development.

Sharing Feelings

When the client's thoughts are clarified, it is helpful to encourage recognition of the feelings associated with the situation. Recognizing feelings and expressing them appropriately will bring a feeling of relief and will allow the client to understand what he or she is experiencing. Feelings can be frightening, and many people are accustomed to ignoring or denying their feelings. The nurse's goal is to give the client permission to share feelings rather than to place demands on him or her when he or she may not

be ready to express emotions. One of the most common emotions observed in clinical settings is sadness and grief. When the nurse notices the client's tearfulness in the context of a situation associated with grief, he or she can hand the client a tissue or touch the client's hand to indicate support. Such an action may be all that is needed to allow the client to begin to cry.

If a client appears ready to cry, the nurse can comment on the behavior in a supportive tone: "You look very sad right now." This sharing of the nurse's observations serves to bring the emotion to the client's attention. The supportive message suggests to the client that the nurse is willing to share the painful feelings. This often results in the client becoming tearful. It is important that the nurse stay with the client until the crying has ended, without trying to prevent expression of the feelings. Being present for someone who is crying can be uncomfortable. The nurse may have the urge to tell the client to stop crying or to give false reassurances, such as "Everything will work out for the best." This has the effect of closing off the expression of emotions. The message is "I do not wish to be burdened with your painful feelings."

In every new situation, clients will experience some degree of anxiety.[2] The tension that results from anxiety will be expressed in behavior such as restlessness or talkativeness. Helping the client to recognize and understand his or her anxiety will be comforting in itself. Comments such as "I notice that you are restless" or "Many people are a bit nervous when they come to the hospital" may help clients pinpoint their own anxiety. If the client believes that being anxious is a sign of weakness, he or she will tend to deny it when asked. Once the nurse conveys that it is acceptable to be anxious, a direct question will often be helpful. Asking "Are you feeling nervous right now?" may then be answered with a "Yes!" This admission of anxiety makes it possible to offer help with relaxation strategies.

Helping the client to express other basic emotions, such as sadness or anger, requires observation on the part of the nurse. The nurse observes for evidence of emotional responses in the client. Clients can be feeling a strong emotion but can be unaware of that emotion at a conscious level. If the nurse confronts the client when he or she is unaware of the feeling, the client may simply deny it. This is frustrating for the nurse and it is not helpful for the client. For example, the nurse observed that Mrs. Bouchard seemed angry. Her facial muscles were tense and her fists were clenched during the description of her daughter's behavior. The nurse asked, "What are you feeling right now?" Mrs. Bouchard answered, "I don't know. I thought we would always be so close, like good friends." When asked about what she was feeling directly, she was unable to put it into words. She told the nurse her thoughts rather than her feelings. To help Mrs. Bouchard express her feelings, the nurse commented about her nonverbal behavior: "I notice that you are clenching your fists when you speak about your daughter. Could it be that you are angry?"

Emotional expression is part of communication, and sharing feelings is a very important supportive function of the nurse. Students sometimes worry that they "caused" the feeling. A comment such as "I made my client cry!" expresses this concern. When clients are sad about the losses they experience, tears may be unexpressed until a supportive person is available to share them. A student who makes him- or herself available may have the privilege of sharing in this powerful human experience.

"Why" Questions

Asking "why?" may seem to be a simple way to gain an understanding of a client's problems, but "why?" is actually very difficult to answer truthfully. Questions that begin with "why?" are confrontational and often put the client on the defensive. With a "why?" question, you are asking the client to do something that is at the least uncomfortable and may even be impossible, which is to explain or defend his or her actions or beliefs. Such a question can interfere with the development of a therapeutic relationship and is never considered therapeutic.

Multiple Questions

Ask only one question at a time. Although this seems obvious, nurses and nursing students often ask two or more questions without pausing for an answer. Under these conditions, the client may react with anxiety as well and be less likely to respond at all. At best, he or she can only answer one question at a time.

SILENCE

Sometimes words are not necessary and silence can express support. Silence is very effective in facilitating communication when the client is having difficulty expressing his or her thoughts. The nurse's willingness to wait quietly demonstrates patience and acceptance. Silence is also effective when the client is struggling to express feelings. Nurses are often surprised at how grateful clients feel when the nurse remains with them in silence while they express strong emotions.

The use of silence is uncommon in social interactions and may take practice before the nurse becomes comfortable with it. It may feel like you are not "doing enough" while staying quietly with a client. Time may seem to pass slowly. Becoming comfortable with the use of silence may be difficult, but the rewards are great.

THERAPEUTIC COMMUNICATION STRATEGIES

Certain techniques that foster or facilitate communication can be learned (Table 4-1). When these techniques are used within the guidelines discussed previously, they can be helpful in the development of a therapeutic relationship.

BARRIERS TO COMMUNICATION

A common barrier to communication is a client's limited use of the English language. It is not uncommon to provide care to clients whose primary language is not English. The client may converse in social situations in English but be unfamiliar with medical terminology. In order to be sure you have an accurate health assessment and can communicate important information, such as discharge teaching, an interpreter is necessary.[3] Another issue arises when the nurse's primary language is not English. Speaking to coworkers or others around you in a language that the client does not understand isolates the client and interferes with the therapeutic relationship. In addition, the client may understand a comment that you did not wish to be heard and understood.

Table 4-1

COMMUNICATION TECHNIQUES: THERAPEUTIC STRATEGIES

Therapeutic Strategy	*Definition*	*Example*
Sharing observations	The nurse shares his or her perceptions with the client	"I notice that you are very talkative today."
General leads	Encouraging the client to continue speaking	"Go on," "Uh-huh," "Really," "Okay."
Identifying themes	The nurse shares consistent topics or issues that arise in the client's conversation	"I notice that your disappointment about your son keeps coming up."
Focusing	Asking the client to elaborate on a specific topic	"I would like to hear more about your sleep difficulties."
Voicing doubt	Expressing gentle disbelief to avoid reinforcing the client's misperceptions	The client tells the nurse that her daughter doesn't care about her feelings. The nurse responds, "Really?"
Presenting reality	The nurse presents his or her view of reality	"I know you think the staff is trying to poison you, but I don't believe that it's true."

The use of jargon is also common in health care settings and can also confuse and isolate the client. Turning to a group of colleagues to discuss the client's situation in technical terms undermines the client's ability to participate in the interaction and demonstrates a lack of regard for his or her dignity and autonomy.

Avoid sounding "all knowing," such as saying "I know just how you feel." These false statements do not reassure the client and lead to mistrust since they are obviously not truthful. They convey the message that you do not have to listen since you already know. Additional examples of nontherapeutic communication are shown in Table 4-2.

DIFFICULT INTERACTIONS WITH CLIENTS

As nurses, we sometimes find ourselves in situations with clients who are uncomfortable. This is the ideal time to seek supervision from a faculty member if you are a student or an experienced clinician if you are a practicing nurse. An objective view can make the difference between a pleasant learning experience and a painful one (Table 4-3).

CONVEYING UPSETTING INFORMATION

One of the most challenging types of communication for nurses is reporting distressing information to the client. It may be as simple as having to tell the client that he will not be going home for the weekend although he was looking forward to it with great anticipation. Or it may be that a family member has called to cancel her long-awaited visit. What these situations have in common is they evoke a feeling of loss. Knowing this in advance will allow the nurse to prepare for expressions of anger and grief. Providing support and allowing the client sufficient time to express the emotions that accompany loss is part of the process of conveying unwelcome information.

Table 4-2

COMMUNICATION TECHNIQUES: NONTHERAPEUTIC STRATEGIES

Nontherapeutic Strategy	Definition	Example
Giving approval	Judging the client by suggesting that he or she did the "right" thing	"I'm proud of the way you stood up to your husband in the family meeting."
Giving disapproval	Judging the client by suggesting that he or she did the "wrong" thing	"Getting up at noon isn't going to help your depression."
Minimizing	Suggesting the client's experience is unimportant	"I wouldn't worry about it. Everyone goes through that."
Changing the subject	Refusing to follow the client's lead in conversation	"Let's talk about something more pleasant."

Table 4-3

DIFFICULT INTERACTIONS

Situation	Example	Therapeutic Response
Client asks for personal information	"I would like your phone number/home address so that I can keep in touch after I go home."	"I'm sorry, but I cannot give my phone number/home address. Are you concerned that you will not be able to reach a team member once you go home?"
	"Do you have children?"	"Yes. Tell me about your family."
Client offers gift	"You have been so good to me. I want you to have this." (Offers money.)	"I appreciate the thought, but I cannot accept it. I enjoyed getting to know you."
Client asks for a favor	"I haven't been out in so long. Will you pick up a few things for me at the store? I'll give you some money."	"I am here to help you with your health problems. I'd like to understand what happened before you came into the hospital."
Client refuses to talk to you	"Please go away. I don't want to talk."	"I will be available to talk with you from 10:00 am to 10:30 am today. I will be sitting in the chair right over there."

Nurses will often be in a position to talk with clients and families in crisis during serious illness, tragic situations, and major life events such as birth and death. What the nurse says and how it is communicated can facilitate acceptance and will often be remembered long after other details of the situation are forgotten. Was the nurse supportive? Caring? Did he or she take time to be with the client and show interest in his or her situation?

How can we communicate frightening, sad, or discouraging information in the most constructive manner possible and encourage questions and further discussion?

Radziewicz and Baile[4] outline a six-step process, SPIKES, for communicating in these situations: S-setting, P-perception, I-invitation, K-knowledge, E-emotions, and S-summary.

The *setting* for such important communication should be private and comfortable. Create an atmosphere in which the client will be comfortable expressing emotions. Include individuals whom the client would like to have around for support. It is easier when those involved get the same information at the same time. They can help one another remember and understand what was said. A transition statement, such as "The news is not as good as we had hoped," helps to prepare the client for what is to come.

Perception refers to what the client and supportive others already understand about the situation. Knowing what they already know allows the nurse to uncover misinformation and to build on what they already understand. The nurse may be surprised to find that the client already has at least some knowledge about the situation.

Invitation involves finding out how much the client wants to know at that time or how much information he or she is ready to take. in. "Would you like me to explain more about what happened?"

Knowledge is introduced slowly while assessing the client's ability to cope with the information. If an individual is not ready to cope with frightening information, he or she may use one of several methods to defend against overpowering anxiety. The client may seem to not "hear" the information, may deny it, or may seem to forget the information soon after it is conveyed. For some, denial may last a few minutes or hours; for others, it may last days or weeks. With time, denial usually gives way to

awareness as the client seeks the opportunity to discuss fears with a supportive person. Denial protects the individual from severe discomfort. Defenses must not be confronted but allowed to operate while they are needed. The nurse can help the client to recognize and talk about fears and misunderstandings. With support and opportunity to talk, most individuals will gradually come to terms with upsetting information. If the client shows no progress toward accepting the reality of the situation, a referral for additional counseling is advisable.

Sometimes family members insist that the client **not** be told difficult news, such as a diagnosis or test results. They usually have the interests of the client at heart and fear that the news is too painful for the client to bear or will result in depression or "giving up." Family members need to know that withholding information will eventually result in the client feeling isolated and sensing that something is wrong.

When the information is received, be prepared for strong *emotions* and remain calm. Let the client know through your words and actions that you are trying to understand his or her feelings. Help the client to express feelings clearly and to use constructive coping strategies. This is a time when empathy is important for the client to believe that you care about the situation.

Anger is a common reaction. It is important to remember that the client is not angry at you but at the situation, and that anger covers up anxiety and disappointment. If you can help the individual express his or her underlying feelings, anger may be diffused. The anger may take the form of blaming you or complaints about care in general. It may be difficult to avoid taking these complaints personally or defending oneself from what seems like a verbal attack. If the individual or significant other feels accepted and comforted, the complaints often decrease or disappear entirely. If the client has a history of violence, alert other staff members that they should be available if needed. Let the client know that you will not allow him or her to hurt him- or herself or others. Set limits on destructive behavior. Let the client know that being destructive with property is not acceptable.

The *summary* is an opportunity to briefly review important information that has been conveyed and to discuss follow-up or what steps need to be taken next. It is important to communicate that there is always hope. Hope may not involve a cure and the nurse cannot reverse the negative events, but it may be possible to assure the client that everything possible will be done to promote his or her comfort and to support his or her choices at this difficult time.

CONCLUSION

Guiding clients through major life experiences such as illness and death is both rewarding and challenging. As you engage in challenging therapeutic interactions, you may wonder if you said the "right" thing. There are no absolute "right" and "wrong" ways to communicate. With supervision and reflection, we can also improve our communication skills. Accepting ourselves and our desire to learn and improve is as important as accepting our clients.

REFERENCES

1. Kotecki CN. Baccalaureate nursing students' communication process in the clinical setting. *J Nurs Educ.* 2002;41(2):61-68.

2. Peplau HE. *Interpersonal Relations in Nursing.* New York: Putnam; 1952.

3. Enslein J, Tripp-Reimer T, Kelley LS, Choi E, McCarty L. Evidence-based protocol: interpreter facilitation for individuals with limited English proficiency. *J Geron Nurs.* 2002;28(7):5-13.

4. Radziewicz R, Baile WF. Communication skills: breaking bad news in the clinical setting. *Oncology Nursing Forum.* 2001;28(6):951-953.

EXERCISES

1. Beginning the Interaction

Opening the conversation requires the use of broad statements or questions that give the client some direction but allows the client freedom to tell his or her "story." Practice writing broad openings as requested below.

>Client: "I'm here because my sister told me to talk to you about the problems I'm having with my husband. I don't see how it will help."
>
>Broad opening from you:

2. Asking for Description

Descriptive questions begin with the words "Who," "What," "Where," and "When." Practice writing descriptive questions as requested below.

>Client: "They told me I had to be admitted to the hospital, but I just want to go home. I felt like hurting myself this morning, but I don't feel that way now."
>
>Descriptive questions from you:

3. Open- and Closed-Ended Questions and Statements

Open-ended questions (or statements) cannot be answered with just one word and are more likely to provide rich descriptions from your client. Closed-ended questions can be answered with one word, such as "yes" or "no," and often lead to little or no elaboration by the client. Practice writing open-ended questions and statements by rewording each of the closed-ended questions that follow.

>Close-ended: "How many children do you have?"
>Open-ended: "Tell me about your family."
>
>Closed-ended: "Do you think the surgery will help?"
>Open-ended:
>
>Closed-ended: "Are you sure you understand the instructions on how to take your medications?"
>Open-ended:
>
>Closed-ended: "Do you think you have a drinking problem?"
>Open-ended:

4. Therapeutic Communication Techniques

Complete the following table with a specific example of the communication technique requested.

THERAPEUTIC COMMUNICATION TECHNIQUES		
Therapeutic Strategy	*Client Behavior*	*Your Therapeutic Response*
Sharing observations	The client crosses and uncrosses her legs repeatedly during the interview.	"I see that you are restless today. I wonder what is going on?"
General leads	"I think I am dying."	
Identifying themes	The client brings up several arguments with her adolescent son.	
Focusing	Mrs. McArthur, a mother of a 2-year-old, comes to the emergency room because her child has been hurt. After 5 minutes of conversation, you are still not sure how the injury happened.	
Voicing doubt	Based on the physical assessment of her child, Mrs. McArthur's explanation of the child's injuries sounds very unlikely.	
Presenting reality	You present your view of the situation with Mrs. McArthur and her child.	

Cross-Cultural Communication

Tamika R. Sanchez-Jones, RN, C, MBA, PhD(c)

OBJECTIVES

1. To discuss the importance of communication with diverse populations
2. To examine cultural differences in communication
3. To describe barriers to cross-cultural communication
4. To describe cultural differences in verbal and nonverbal communication
5. To examine individual cultural backgrounds and influence on health care beliefs, values, and behavior
6. To discuss the use of bilingual interpreters to reduce the effects of language barriers

The ability to effectively send and receive messages is essential to communication and allows individuals to interact with one another. This interaction may be especially difficult when the sender and receiver do not share the same cultural background or language. Culture influences how each individual perceives and responds to the world, solves life's problems, and interacts with others. Although there is no single definition of culture, culture may be defined as the sum total of behavioral norms, methods of communication, patterns of thinking, beliefs, and values of a designated group of people. These can be passed down to the next generation. This may

be evident in day-to-day interactions. When shopping or engaging in social activities you may encounter people who shop in the same stores or wear the same clothes, but who look and talk differently than you. During these interactions, regardless of how brief, there may be awareness of the influence of culture on communication. Differences in communication across cultures are evident in language, verbal and nonverbal behaviors, and silence.[1]

Why is culture significant to nursing? Recent demographic trends indicate increasing cultural and ethnic diversity in the United States, leading to a more diverse client population. Within the health care setting, nurses and other providers understand the importance of communication when working with clients. However, there is less understanding of the impact of culture on the communication process. Nurses spend a great deal of their time with clients and, therefore, must realize the importance of culture as it relates to communication. Transcultural nursing skills and knowledge will be necessary to provide competent care to the rapidly changing, heterogeneous population.

Learning to value cultural and ethnic diversity involves the appreciation of variations in culture as well as negotiating skills for effective communication. Communication with individuals from diverse backgrounds is especially complex because of the

---

Table 5-1

GUIDELINES FOR CROSS-CULTURAL COMMUNICATION

Do

* Be aware of your own cultural beliefs and biases
* Be open to learning more about others' communication styles
* Practice engaging in cross-cultural communication
* Listen actively and allow time for cross-cultural communication
* Respect others' decisions to engage in communication with you
* Explore speech patterns of cultural groups
* Be aware of nonverbal communication
* Clarify messages
* Be aware that communication occurs in context

Do Not

* Stereotype
* Assume there is only one way to communicate (yours)
* Assume that breakdowns in communication are due to others' errors
* Presume communication means understanding
* Assume all cultures are similar to yours

Adapted from Smith-Trudeau P. Communication guarantees nothing. *Vermont Nurse Connection.* 2001;4(4):1,3.

---

influence of culture on language and communication. When communicating with individuals, the nurse should be aware of cultural beliefs and behaviors, and communicate (both verbally and nonverbally) in a way that meets the clients' cultural needs. Meeting the needs of clients requires the ability to provide and understand clear and accurate communication.

Intercultural or cross-cultural communication refers to the presence of at least two individuals who are culturally different from each other on important attributes such as value orientations, preferred communication codes, role expectations, and perceived rules of social relationships.[2] In intercultural communication, differences in communication styles are often met with confusion, impatience, and misunderstanding. Imagine how difficult it would be to communicate when the listener does not share the same language, context, or symbolism. How could you teach a newly diagnosed insulin-dependent diabetic about dietary management and medication regimens when there is not a shared language or culture? How could you assist in developing menu plans when you are unaware of culturally specific foods? How could you explain the use of insulin and the procedure for administration if you do not speak the language?

These issues represent the difficulties in intercultural communication. Table 5-1 offers guidelines for cross-cultural communication.

Although knowledge of cultural rules and norms can help to avoid mistakes in communication, it is not possible for individuals to be familiar or competent with the differences in communication patterns for all cultures. Even when aware of cultural differences, it is difficult to consider the subtle differences among individuals within the same culture. Nurses must be open to subgroup variability within cultures. Differences may be seen within the culture based on factors such as gender, educational level, income, and status.

OVERCOMING BARRIERS TO PROVIDING CROSS-CULTURAL CARE

When caring for clients from diverse populations, nurses should be aware of their own cultural behaviors and habits. Each individual is socialized into a cultural environment. Assuming cultures are similar to your own will lead to confusion and misinterpretation of messages. It is better to expect differences and explore ways in which these differences will affect communication. Nurses may have little awareness of how their own cultural beliefs define the type of care they give or messages they send to clients. Both nonverbal and verbal communication skills are important in the nursing process. How would a client from a different culture respond to personal questions regarding health practices or personal history? How do others perceive personal uses of distance, gestures, and dialect? Cultural differences in both verbal and nonverbal communication will be discussed later in this chapter.

Cultural barriers may also be present in the way in which members of an ethnic group perceive health, illness, and discharge following treatment.[3] For example, clients who view illness as a punishment or curse may delay medical treatment or seek medical treatment only as a last resort. Respect for cultural traditions will take into account alternative health care practices and beliefs, such as the use of lay practitioners and complementary therapies while incorporating medical interventions.

Ethnocentric values may make it difficult for the nurse to be objective in providing care, especially to diverse populations. Ethnocentrism is the belief that one's own culture is superior to that of another.[4] Being proud of one's own culture is appropriate, but the difficulty begins when there is less respect for the values or beliefs outside of one's own. For example, instead of trying to understand a newly admitted client from the client's cultural context, the ethnocentric nurse would try to understand the client within the nurse's own cultural context. Nurses should respect the differences in behavior and knowledge that may influence health care practices and recognize that their own ideas or behaviors may not be best for every client.[5] Ethnocentrism may make it difficult for the nurse to accept client decisions not based on the nurse's culturally derived value system or beliefs.

Case Example

Mr. Rodriquez, a 65-year-old Hispanic male, was admitted to the hospital at 8 pm following a stroke. Visiting hours were just ending, and Mr. Rodriquez was accompanied by his wife and four grown children and their spouses. The nurse felt overwhelmed with so many relatives present, but they were insistent that they needed to stay with the client through the night. What would be the nurse's most appropriate course of action?

HIGH- AND LOW-CONTEXT CULTURES

Hall[6] conceptualized high- and low-context cultures. When individuals attempt to communicate, it is important to understand the amount of information transmitted through words vs the context of the situation. Context refers to the situation and/or environment where the communication occurs and helps to define the communication. Culture is also considered context and may set the stage for communication. However, cultures may differ in the amount and type of information conveyed through verbal and nonverbal cues.

In intercultural interactions, there are differences in high- and low-context communication patterns. Individuals from *high-context* cultures rely on an understanding of shared experiences without the need for many words. There is meaning attached to the context, and there is more communication contained in the context of the situation vs the words spoken. Emphasis is placed on nonverbal interactions such as nonverbal cues and messages.[7,8] Ideas are being communicated through eye contact, facial expressions, body posture, and perceptions of personal space. People from high-context cultures consider themselves part of the larger group and value shared experiences. There is also an appreciation for history and tradition. One example of high-context culture is likely your own family environment. When communicating with individuals with whom you are familiar, such as family members, there is little need for explanations or highly detailed information. In high-context cultures, there is a familiarity with one another, and minimal verbal communication is needed to gain understanding. In these situations, even facial expressions can communicate complex messages. There is an underlying message or metaphoric association in the communication.[9] For example, you probably knew your mother was displeased by your behavior with just "a look," or you can signal approval of a friend's new outfit with a wink or the "thumbs up sign." There is little need for your mother to give you a detailed explanation of her disapproval of your behavior, and a friend would clearly understand your nonverbal communication without the need for clarification. Asians, Saudi Arabians, Spaniards, Africans, African Americans, and Native Americans engage in high-context communication.

In the case example, the nurse recognized that Mr. Rodriquez is part of a high-context cultural group and understood the value he places on being part of a group and sharing important experiences with the group. Nonverbal communication is facilitated when family members are present. In this situation, the nurse would be creative and flexible about including family members while respecting the needs of other clients.

Cultures that engage in *low-context* communication use more words and are impatient with others who do not make themselves understood quickly. Meaning is derived from the message. There is less meaning attached to the context. Verbal messages are elaborate, highly detailed, and redundant. Low-context cultures lack shared meanings and continuity. The ability to make oneself understood is valued. Individuals from low-context cultures may not understand the use of gestures and nonverbal cues frequently used in high-context cultures.[7] Low-context communication is best described by the type of communication one would have with a stranger in which you would have to explain ideas in detail because there may be no shared understanding or experiences. Silence and other nonverbal cues may be confusing and irritating to low-context communicators. Those from low-context cultures include Anglo-Europeans, Canadians, Americans, and Germans.

When communication is attempted between individuals from a high-context and those from a low-context culture, the high-context communicator offers little information or clarity and utilizes silence and nonverbal cues to encourage understanding. This may be very frustrating to those from a low-context culture. In contrast, the low-context communicator offers elaborate explanations, which may lead the high-context communicator to believe that he or she is not being understood. When high-context communicators receive a detailed response, they surmise that their message was ignored or missed.

VERBAL COMMUNICATION

Communication Patterns

Not only do we base our opinions of others on verbal communication, but we also attempt to define social status and emotions on the way a person speaks and makes him- or herself understood. Communication patterns, pitch, and rate differ among cultures. African Americans share and express feelings openly to family members and close friends. The pitch may be fast and the tone loud and confrontational. For European Americans, the pitch is slower and the tone is less challenging and less personal. Asians are typically soft-spoken and do not challenge during conversation. Muslim or Arabic speech tends to be repetitive and exaggerated. Displays of emotion represent a deep concern for the topic of discussion.

The discussion of personal issues with strangers is considered inappropriate within the African American, Arabian, and Asian cultures. In contrast, Latinos will usually appreciate inquiries about family members. In the health care setting, variations in verbal communication may be evident while trying to take a health history or attempting to understand the religious practices of an African American client. African Americans believe in prayer to promote health and well-being. African Americans may also "speak in tongues," a prayer which is understood only by the person speaking; therefore, this display of prayer and spirituality may be confusing for individuals from other cultures. Asians, Middle Easterners, and Latin Americans seek to "save face" at all costs. The dignity of these clients must be preserved at all times to avoid "loss of face." Nurses need to be particularly sensitive to avoid humiliation or inadvertent slights within these cultures.[10]

Regional, racial, and ethnic accents are also important and may lead to assumptions or stereotyping. The accents and speech patterns of urban minority youths may be perceived negatively by educated Anglo-Europeans. What other types of accents or regional dialects can you identify that are associated with strong assumptions?

NONVERBAL COMMUNICATION

It is often said that "actions speak louder than words," and this may be especially true when communicating across cultures. Nonverbal communication can be defined as the deliberate or non-intentional use of touch, distance, space, gestures, and time to communicate meaning. These messages may indicate approval, status, emotion, and power. Effective communication considers not only the spoken word but also the nonverbal nuances.

Additional forms of nonverbal communication not discussed in this chapter include email, clothing, tattoos, and artifacts (physical objects such as cars, jewelry, etc).

Touch

Touch is a meaningful form of nonverbal communication.[11] The amount and type of touch may differ related to gender, age, socioeconomic factors, and individual preferences.[7] Touch can indicate emotions from approval and comfort to aggression and anger. For example, patting someone on the back can indicate approval or acceptance in many cultures, while touching someone with the left hand is considered inappropriate and disrespectful among Muslims. In addition, for strict Muslims and Orthodox Jews, a handshake between men and women in a public setting is inappropriate and considered disrespectful.

Mexican and Native Americans believe that touch is magical and healing. Within the Vietnamese culture, touch may provoke anxiety because it is thought to release the soul from the body.[5] Touching the head, even of a small child, may be viewed as offensive to some Asians. African Americans and Hispanics tend to be comfortable with close personal space and frequently touch while interacting with close friends and relatives.

Handshaking is a generally accepted greeting in America, especially in business. The type and length of a handshake differs across cultures. In America, the handshake is firm. In Asia, the handshake is soft with the other hand brought up underneath to signify warmth and friendship. In contrast, many Latin Americans view the handshake as impersonal and distant.

Culture influences the amount and type of physical contact that is considered acceptable. It is usually a good idea to ask questions and explain the reason for touch, such as physical examination, prior to initiating the touch. Be open to feedback and adapt your behavior as necessary.

Personal Space

The amount of distance and space between yourself and the client highly influences the message sent. The amount of acceptable space differs among cultures and may also vary within cultures based on gender and other variables. Familiarity and trust may also determine the comfortable distance. Regardless of cultural background, we each have some sense of comfortable distance and feel uncomfortable when others are "in our space." Are there people who you can identify that make you uncomfortable because they invade your space? Do you notice that people often step backward or step into you when you are attempting to communicate?

The nature of relationships is conveyed through the use of personal zones. Hall[12] defines extensions of personal space across cultures, and the following zones define these distances.

* **Intimate zone (touching):** 18 inches; occurs during private situations. This distance is best for assessing breath and body odors. When this space is invaded by someone other than those who are emotionally close, we feel threatened. Visual distortions also occur in this zone, and the voice may be at a whisper.
* **Personal zone:** 18 inches to 4 feet; occurs most often as the distance during a handshake. It is also the distance most couples stand in public. The voice is moderate, body odor is not apparent, and there are no physical distortions. The physical examination typically occurs at this distance.
* **Social/casual zone:** 4 to 8 feet; occurs during impersonal business transactions. Interviews occur at this distance.
* **Public zone:** Beyond 8 feet; occurs in situations such as teaching and other less personal interactions. The speaker must project his or her voice and it is difficult to assess facial expression due to distance.

Hispanics and Asians typically prefer less distance and stand closer to each other than do Anglo-Europeans. The nurse should also be aware that many cultures prefer that same-sex health care providers perform intimate physical and mental examinations. The nurse should try to meet the client's request to preserve modesty and participation.

When working with clients who prefer more personal space, the nurse may sit in a chair at the end of the bed in an acute care setting or in a chair opposite the client in a community or clinic setting. When less distance is desired, the nurse may sit at the head of the bed or closer to the client.

Gestures

Gestures can also communicate messages and cues to others. Expressions of self through body movements can facilitate and enhance communication.

Head nodding, pointing, smiles, and general body movements can help to clarify other forms of communication. These vary among cultures. In a number of cultures, nodding of the head signifies agreement. However, within the Japanese culture head nodding is indicative of attentiveness, not agreement, and could be easily misunderstood.[13] Pointing, as in summoning a waiter, is commonplace in American society, while in other cultures it is considered rude.

Emotions may also be influenced by culture. While Americans may openly laugh or smile when happy or amused, Asians may laugh or smile when speaking of unpleasant or embarrassing situations. Koreans, in contrast, believe that laughing and frequent smiling demonstrate unintelligence and, therefore, are often serious under most circumstances.

Eye Contact

Patterns of eye contact differ across cultures. Eye contact communicates respect, status, and regulates turn-taking in a conversation in American society. In American society, one may look away or avoid direct eye contact when one is embarrassed or uncomfortable in a situation. Think back to a time when you may have avoided direct eye contact when a professor posed a question for which you did not know the answer.

A direct stare by African Americans or Arabians is not intended as a threat or a sign of rudeness, while an indirect or downward gaze is seen as a sign of respect among most Asians.

TIME

Attempting to communicate across cultural barriers requires knowledge by the nurse of the differences in the perception of time. Have you ever noticed how some people are always late regardless of the situation, while others are punctual to a fault? The perception of time varies among cultures. Time orientation determines if members of a cultural group view time in the present, past, or future. Cultures that are future oriented plan long-term and are readily accepting of health care regimens to prevent future illness. They keep appointments more often and engage in health promotion activities. Clients who are oriented to the present show less concern for health care regimens and are less likely to keep or be on time for appointments.[1] A shared belief by African Americans and Mexican Americans is that time is flexible and that events do not begin until they arrive. The nurse who is aware of this cultural variation will allow some flexibility when planning care for these clients.

UTILIZING BILINGUAL TRANSLATORS

There may be situations when you must confront differences in both culture and language. This may become very difficult in explaining a diagnosis or trying to obtain informed consent for a medical treatment. Although most health care institutions offer some type of service and/or provide staff to meet the needs of culturally diverse patients, nurses can be effective in preparing themselves for the interaction. Using interpreters can assist nurses in communication across language barriers. When there are no formally trained interpreters available, a bilingual family member may serve as an interpreter.

While it may be convenient to use family members, clients may also be less willing to disclose personal information and therefore make the nurse-client relationship difficult and awkward. Often children are used to interpret because they are usually more proficient in the second language. Parents, children, or close friends and family members may be reluctant to share personal or intimate matters because of embarrassment. It is particularly awkward for a child to ask a parent personal health information, and it may be equally discomforting for a parent to reveal such information to a child interpreter. Family members may also have limited knowledge of the content needed to adequately relate health information and provide medical direction. Due to the sensitive issues often discussed in the nurse-client relationship, the use of children as interpreters is discouraged. When possible, the use of professionally trained, same-sex interpreters is preferred. In addition, it is recommended that the nurse meet with the interpreter to review the goals and purposes of meeting with the family. It is also a good idea for the interpreter to meet with the family to prepare for the session as well as establish rapport. The nurse should speak directly to the client and family during the session and not to the interpreter. Avoiding complicating medical jargon and keeping answers simple and concrete help to avoid mishaps in translation. Also allow plenty of time for the interpreter to relay information and encourage questions when appropriate. The use of good interpreters is an invaluable resource to nurses and the health care team.[14]

CONCLUSION

The ability to communicate, both verbally and nonverbally, to diverse populations is crucial to providing effective transcultural care. A culturally sensitive nurse seeks to incorporate knowledge of the client's culture in providing therapeutic nursing care. Lack of effective communication may impede the nursing process when working with diverse clients. Cultural and language differences do not need to pose barriers to providing nursing care. The greater your understanding of communication patterns of diverse cultures, the more effective your ability to communicate. Practice and more practice are essential to increase competence in cross-cultural communication.

REFERENCES

1. Spector RE. *Cultural Diversity in Health and Illness*. 5th ed. Saddle Ridge, NJ: Prentice Hall Health; 2000.

2. Lustig MW, Koester J. *Intercultural Competence*. New York: Addison Wesley; 1998.

3. Betchel GA, Davidhizar R. A cultural assessment model for ED patients. *Journal of Emergency Nursing*. 2002;25(5):377-380.

4. Leininger MM. *Cultural Care Diversity & Universitality. A Theory of Nursing*. New York: National League for Nursing; 1991.

5. Giger JN, Davidhizar RE. *Transcultural Nursing. Assessment and Intervention*. 3rd ed. St. Louis: Mosby; 1995.

6. Hall ET. *Beyond Culture*. New York: Doubleday; 1976.

7. Lynch EW, Hanson MJ. *Developing Cross-Cultural Competence: A Guide for Working With Children and Their Families*. 2nd ed. Baltimore: Paul H. Brooks; 1998.

8. Harris PR, Moran RT. *Managing Cultural Differences: Leadership Strategies for a New World of Business*. Houston, Tex: Gulf Pub; 2000.

9. Kabagarama D. *Breaking the Ice: A Guide to Understanding People From Other Cultures*. Boston: Allyn and Bacon; 1993.

10. Gardenswartz L, Rowe A. *Managing Diversity in Health Care*. San Francisco: Jossey-Bass; 1998.

11. DeFleur ML, Kearney P, Plax TG. *Fundamentals of Human Communication*. Mountain View, Calif: Mayfield; 1993.

12. Hall ET. *The Silent Language*. New York: Doubleday; 1959.

13. Lum D. *Social Work Practice and People of Color: A Process-Stage Approach*. Monterey, Calif: Brooks/Cole; 1996.

14. Enslein J, Tripp-Reimer T, Kelley LS, Choi E, McCarty L. Evidence-based protocol: interpreter facilitation for individuals with limited English proficiency. *J Geron Nurs*. 2002;28(7):5-13.

EXERCISES

1. Self-Assessment

Review and answer each question independently, then compare your answers with someone within your family and discuss with a group of friends or colleagues.

* When you were a child, what were the health care beliefs and behaviors of your family?

* What did your family do to stay healthy?

* What did your family believe caused illness?

* How were specific illnesses treated?

* Who was responsible for deciding the appropriate treatment?

* What health care practitioners outside of the family were used to treat illness?

A. How are the answers to the questions similar and/or different from your family members' answers?

B. How are the answers to the questions similar and/or different from your friends' or colleagues' answers?

C. What surprised you the most while completing this exercise?

2. Beliefs About Diverse Cultural Groups

Examine your personal beliefs about the following cultural groups. How might your personal beliefs and values affect your ability to communicate with individuals from each of the cultural groups? You may choose to do this privately so that you may be honest with your answers.

✳ Mexican Americans

✳ Africans

✳ Chinese Americans

✳ Japanese Americans

✳ European Americans

✳ Cuban Americans

✳ African Americans

✳ Navajos

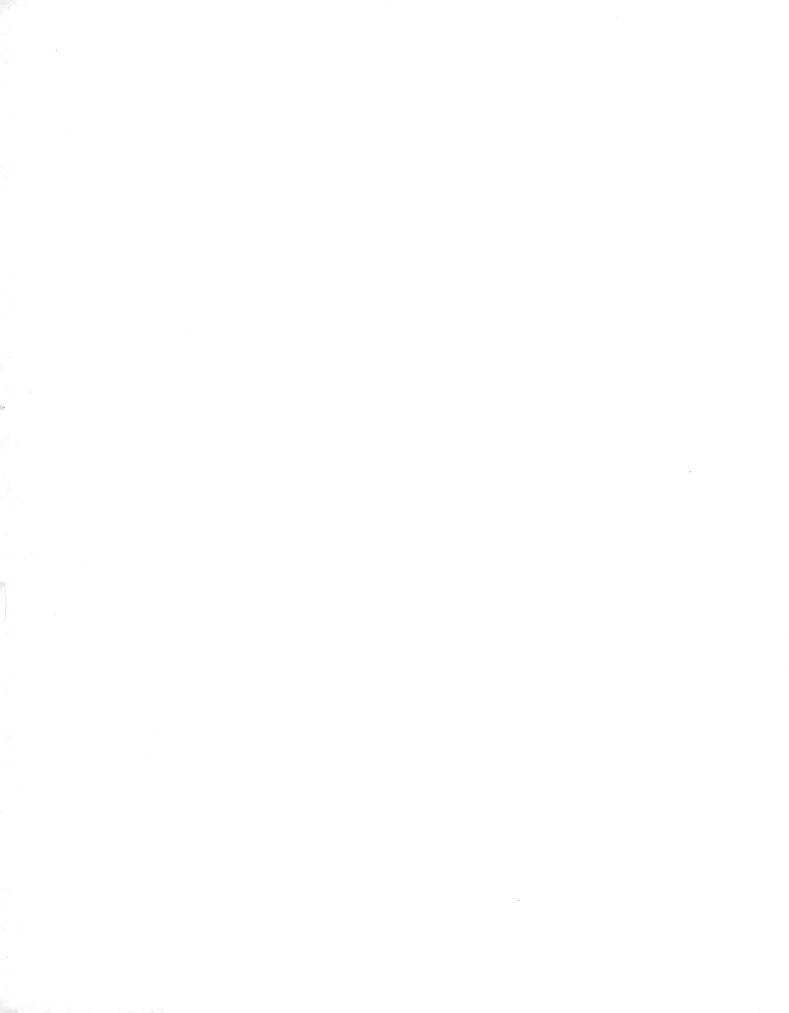

SECTION

III

Communicating in Special Circumstances

Communicating With Children

Lois S. Marshall, PhD, RN, CPN

OBJECTIVES

1. To describe the development of language as a means of communication
2. To discuss normal communication patterns of children of various ages
3. To discuss strategies that the nurse can use to enhance communication with children

INTRODUCTION

Once upon a time, a small rabbit was lost in a maze. The rabbit searched and circled looking for a way to his destination. During the trip, the rabbit came across a giraffe. The rabbit came up to the giraffe's big toenail. The giraffe asked the rabbit if help was needed. The rabbit looked up tentatively and somewhat awed with the size of the giraffe. The rabbit took two steps backward and looked up... way up... way, way up. With trepidation, the rabbit said, "No, thank you," and started to move away.

Such is the communication between children and nurses who tower over them. Nurses look different than children, just as the giraffe looks different from the rabbit. The differences in appearance, size, and development will affect the communication patterns between nurses and children. These differences must be addressed to better understand normal communication patterns of children of different ages and cognitive levels. For nurses to communicate with children effectively, the rabbit and giraffe scenario must be avoided by adapting communication techniques to the appropriate level of the children they are caring for.

FAMILY-CENTERED COMMUNICATION

Communication with children is family centered. It is a process involving the nurse, parent(s) or caregiver, and child.[1] In today's society of expanded and nontraditional families, there may be many other participants in the communication process, and nurses should note that the principles of communication with families are the same regardless of family make-up.

Although nurses must communicate with both the child and family members to be effective as health care providers, the age and cognitive development of the child dictate how much communication will take place with all members of the family present and when separate discussions might be more appropriate. Nurses working with children must have knowledge of family dynamics, relationships, cultural differences, and established communication patterns within the family structure. It is knowledge of how the family communicates that will best assist the nurse in determining the ideal strategy for communicating with the child separately and as an active, participating member of the family.

COMMUNICATION IN CHILDREN

For children, communication is a process that evolves as cognition, physical and psychosocial development, and experience increase. Communication takes practice and repetition, interaction with role models, confidence, as well as verbal and nonverbal skills. As early as gestation, humans participate in varying forms of communication. Prospective parents listen to classical music, talk to their baby, and read books to "mommy's tummy" in hopes that these forms of language are heard, even at a very basic level.

From infancy through adolescence, communication is a dynamic, ongoing, ever-changing, and constantly developing process. Communication continues as the infant begins to interact with the environment and the people in it. Somatic language[2] is primarily the language of infants' communication, although components of this means of communication can continue throughout one's lifespan. Somatic language is focused on communicating through nonverbal vocalization, such as crying to make an infant's needs heard; facial expressions, as when an infant grimaces and spits out a new food that tastes bad; jerking movements; and the reddening of skin, as in frustration in an infant, which in later life is often identified as blushing with embarrassment. Action language[2] begins later in infancy, as the child learns to communicate wants and needs by reaching, pointing, crawling toward or away, turning his or her head, and/or closing his or her lips. The infant's ability to communicate is guided by what these actions mean to him- or herself and how these actions are interpreted by the caregiver. Verbal language,[2] while beginning with the first spoken word at 6 to 7 months of age, does not really become an effective means of communication until toddlerhood. The toddler's language development progresses from repetitive noises and sounds to word usage, to phrase usage, and finally to sentence usage. This process grows and becomes more refined with experience and cognitive development throughout one's lifetime.

COMMUNICATION/COGNITIVE DEVELOPMENT

The younger infant, age 1 to 6 months, uses primarily nonverbal communication. The infant responds to adults through tactile stimulation and by the sound and tone of the adult's voice. At this age, the infant uses vocalization on a limited basis through crying and cooing. Nursing strategies appropriate for children at this stage include the use of touch; speaking in a high-pitched, gentle voice; maintaining eye contact with the infant; and using play appropriately (eg, "peekaboo"). The older infant, age 6 to 12 months, builds on what has been learned previously. At this age, the infant is starting to become egocentric (the child sees him- or herself as the center of the universe). The infant is beginning to build a vocabulary, with the first words spoken at 6 to 7 months of age. At this stage, the infant begins to experience "stranger anxiety" (a new behavior that involves withdrawing from or rejecting unfamiliar people) and has no sense of object permanence (when an object is out of sight, it does not exist). Nursing strategies on which to focus include all that were used with the younger infant; in addition, the nurse should look for clues that the infant wants to play or interact, as through eye contact or reaching out with his or her arms.[1]

The toddler/preschool years span a large range, from 1 to 6 years of age. These children remain egocentric and focus on communication for and about themselves, how they feel, and what they can do. Toddlers continue to communicate with their hands when the words are not there. Toddlers and preschoolers are rapidly acquiring language skills, including rapid growth in vocabulary and in the ability to use it in sentences as they reach the preschool years. At this age, the child easily misinterprets phrases and interprets words literally. For example, "coughing your head off" means that your head will fall off of your body, "a little stick in the arm" means a tree stick will be put in the child's arm, and "bleeding out" means blood will come out of the body without stopping. The child is a concrete thinker at this age.

Communication strategies for toddlers includes using patience in listening, as it sometimes takes the child extra time to express his or her thoughts in words. Do not interrupt the child. Do not discuss frightening or serious subjects with the parents in the presence of the child. Choose your words carefully, keeping in mind the possibility of misinterpretations. Set limits for the child in order to provide a sense of security. Offer structured choices and redirect and/or reframe behavior when warranted. For example, the child can be given a choice between two different foods for lunch rather than asking an open-ended question such as "What would you like to eat for lunch?" Using play as a form of communication can enhance the child's ability to tell you what is needed or desired. Age-appropriate play is discussed in greater detail later in this chapter.

The school-age period includes children ages 6 to 12 years old. The child in this age group wants explanations and reasons for everything, such as what procedures are being done to him or her step-by-step and why. The school-age child is an enthusiastic participant in communication who needs relatively simple explanations at the beginning of the stage of development. As the child progresses from thinking concretely early in this age period to more abstract thinking as the end of this period approaches, more complete explanations can be given. A child at this age wants to use logic and often misinterprets adult conversations. Nursing strategies to focus on include using simple, straightforward questions and answers. The school-age child is often reluctant to communicate his or her own needs, so speaking and responding in the third person is useful in communication. For example, the nurse remarks, "Some children like to hold my hand when their IV is started." It is also important for the nurse to obtain the child's perceptions before any explanations are given in order to avoid confusion.

The adolescent period ranges in age from 12 to 18 years. This child fluctuates between child-like and adult thinking and behavior. The adolescent has a genuine interest in the care that is being provided and wants to participate in the decision-making process. As the later teen years approach, the adolescent is caught between wanting to be "grown up" and the security that comes from remaining a child. The adolescent has attitudes and feelings that need to be communicated about a wide range of topics, such as peer groups, identity, sex, substance abuse, and his or her parents. The nurse must recognize where and when to discuss these issues with the adolescent and

how much communication can take place with and without the parents. Communicating with the adolescent begins with the development of trust. It is essential for the nurse to build a rapport with the adolescent, to listen vs talk, and to be nonjudgmental and straightforward. Although you may not approve of some of the adolescent's behavior, it is important to communicate acceptance of the person. The nurse must let the adolescent control the communication within the limitations of confidentiality without minimizing thoughts and feelings.[1,3]

COMMUNICATION STRATEGIES WITH CHILDREN

There are many traditional as well as nontraditional communication techniques that can be very successful with children of all ages. These communication techniques can be delineated as being verbal, nonverbal, or a combination of both. Verbal techniques include word games and storytelling. Nonverbal techniques include drawing and story writing. For example, in order to learn more about the child's family relationships, you could ask the child to draw a picture of him- or herself and family members doing an activity together. Then ask the child to tell you about the drawing. This strategy engages the child in talking about how he or she views his or her family. Combination communication techniques center on various forms of play therapy. Young children will often spontaneously act out their experiences with dolls or plush animals and reveal their feelings and concerns. Communicating with children takes time and patience, thought and skill, creativity and practice, and, of course, a desire to communicate with children in whatever way possible to reach each unique individual.

Table 6-1 lists "do's" and "don'ts" adapted from Boggs'[4] recommendations for establishing rapport with children.

Sydnor-Greenberg and Dokken[5] conducted a study of communication patterns between children and health care providers. They interviewed children ages 4 to 17 and then interviewed the children's mothers separately. Based on their interviews, the researchers developed the "CLEAR" communication framework:

"C" is the context of the communication between the child and the health care provider. The child is more than just a diagnosis or health problem. He or

---

Table 6-1

TIPS FOR EFFECTIVE COMMUNICATION WITH CHILDREN

Do	*Do Not*
✳ Get to know a child's developmental level	✳ Make a child self-conscious by drawing attention to him- or herself
✳ Learn the child's interests based on your observations of his or her activities	✳ Use abstractions with a child who is a concrete thinker (eg, for a child who does not understand time, tell him or her "after lunch" not "later" or "at 2:00 pm")
✳ Talk at the child's level and with vocabulary he or she will understand	
✳ "Level the playing field" by sharing your thoughts and/or observations about what is happening to the child	✳ Jump to conclusions
	✳ Get "in the middle" between a child and a parent, especially in front of the child
✳ Maintain a calm, unhurried, caring, gentle approach	
✳ Use concrete examples and/or link information to activities of daily living vs abstractions	
✳ Allow opinions to be expressed	
✳ Be an active, attentive listener	

Adapted from Boggs K. Communicating with children. In: Arnold E, Boggs K, eds. *Interpersonal Relationships: Professional Communication Skills for Nurses.* 3rd ed. Philadelphia: WB Saunders; 1999.

---

she has a life outside of the illness and wants that to be acknowledged by the health care provider. "L" is for listening to the child, actively listening to what he or she has to say, what he or she does not say, and what he or she needs help saying. Listening is a partnership that requires participation by both the child and the health care provider. "E" is for empowerment. Empowerment implies an active role for the child. Children want to know, to be informed, and to have meaningful input to any communication. Children do not want to be talked about, overlooked, ignored, or "brushed off," as if to say their input is irrelevant and not necessary. "A" stands for advice, providing relevant information to the child. Children want to be taught, want to know what lies ahead, and how they can assist in the management of their care. These data allow the child a certain degree of independence, which he or she would be working toward if he or she were outside the health care environment. "R" stands for reassurance that the child is recovering, healthy, and managing his or her care well. Children do not want false reassurance anymore than adults do; children do not want to be lied to, nor do they want the truth to be omitted completely.

Child-Specific Communication Strategies

The following strategies can be used to better assess the child and to give him or her an opportunity to express any needs.

Word Games

Word games are an effective means of communicating, especially for children who have at least a moderate degree of language development. Word games can include a version of the "happy faces" game, in which the nurse asks the child to describe how his or her face looks today, yesterday, and how it will look tomorrow. The nurse should focus on the words the child uses. Do the words change with the child's perception of health and are the words more positive or negative in tone? Word games can be extended to word association, moving from more neutral words to more anxiety-provoking words. "Describe in one word how you feel." "Sick," "surgery," "hospital," and other words that are specific to the health/illness experience can be used. The nurse needs to remember that word games must be appropriate for the child's age and cognitive and developmental stages.

Storytelling

Storytelling can be guided and/or directed, as in "tell a story about a girl/boy like you" or "tell a story about this picture." Storytelling can also be free, as in "tell about anything you want." Storytelling allows reality and imagination to become integrated. By creating characters in a story, children can express concerns and explore what is happening to them without becoming too personally invested. Storytelling allows the child to communicate in a comfortable way with control over the communication process. The more focused the nurse wants the child to be, the more guidance or direction should be given. The more exploration the nurse wants the child to do, the less guidance and direction the nurse should give. It is important to stress that too much structure can shift the child's communication. The nurse needs to allow the child to dictate the direction of the story. The child needs to be able to be creative, imaginative, and real according to his or her own ability extent and the nurse must then extrapolate the meaning of the story based on clues the child is giving/communicating.

Drawing

Drawing is another means of encouraging a child to express him- or herself without words. It allows the externalization of internal mental images and emotions.[6] Depending on age, drawing is an activity that children often do in the normal course of a day; therefore, it is safe and familiar. When using drawing as a communication technique, the emphasis is not on how well the picture/art is drawn, but in the ability to get in touch with feelings and healing through the drawing. When a child is not verbally sophisticated, drawing can be extremely helpful in facilitating communication. When a child is overwhelmed by experiences, the environment, or the uncertain or unknown, drawing can be therapeutic. The nurse can gain insight into a child who is undergoing painful procedures or experiencing fears, concerns, or problems through the process of drawing.

Drawing can be structured in that the child can be asked to draw something specific about an emotion or experience. Unstructured drawing or asking a child to draw whatever he or she wants is a very effective method to explore feelings and concerns. The child can be encouraged to include written details of the drawn images if he or she so desires. Drawings can be in black and white or include colors. Let the child decide which colors to use, as color is expressive of emotions. Toys, such as a color wand or a color-changing necklace to express mood in color, are available to allow the child to use colors to express him- or herself.[7] Drawings can include symbols as well, again to be determined by the child, rather than the nurse. Drawing as a form of communication can be very effective in facilitating expression of a child's deepest emotions. DiGallo and Netzer-Stein[8] found that drawing allowed children with cancer to express their fears and could also be used to assess a child's ability to cope.

Story Writing

Story writing is similar to storytelling but is used with an older child or adolescent. Story writing can be used to express or communicate feelings, thoughts, beliefs, and/or fears that can be verbally expressed. The writing process can take many forms, from actual event-driven stories, to journal writing, writing letters to an actual person or to oneself, or writing on the Internet. The internet offers several possibilities including email, "chat rooms" or posting a story on a web page. Writing allows personal reflection while maintaining some degree of privacy. Story writing, like storytelling, can be both structured and unstructured. The nurse can be guided by clues from the child as to which actually will accomplish the therapeutic goal most effectively.

Play

Play is children's work. It is what they know, what they understand, and it is how they communicate. In play, children utilize both verbal and nonverbal communication skills to express their feelings without acknowledging cognitively and/or intellectually that they are doing so. Play can be structured or free and can take on many forms depending on the age and cognitive development of the child. Play activities as a form of communication can include simple hand games with an infant, "peekaboo" with an older infant, play with safe medical equipment for the older toddler and preschooler,

---

Case Example

When verbal communication is uncomfortable for a child, for whatever reason, play activities can assist the child in communicating his or her feelings. The following clinical case study illustrates the very important connection between play and communication with a child.

Mark is a 10-year-old boy who was admitted to the hospital with a diagnosis of vesicoureteral reflux and who was scheduled for a surgical repair. Following surgery, Mark had a Foley catheter in place that was to be advanced daily by the urologist. Each morning, the nurse noticed that as the time grew closer to the doctor arriving, Mark's vital signs increased, and he became agitated and diaphoretic. When asked what was wrong or if he wanted to talk, he closed his eyes and pulled the covers up to his chin. One day, the nurse stayed with him as he heard the footsteps of the doctor down the hall. His increased anxiety was consistent with the anticipation of what was to occur—the advancement of his catheter.

Based on the clues Mark had given, the nurse had an idea about an age/developmentally appropriate means of communication that would possibly encourage him to deal with his feelings about the threatening situation he was experiencing. The nurse took a pillowcase and stuffed it with filling, then tied it at the end. She took it to Mark with a big black marker and told him the pillow was his to do with as he wished. He drew the face of the doctor on it and he even put the doctor's name on top. The nurse put a hook through the top and connected it to the patient drape rod that encircled the room. She placed the "doc" in front of Mark and left him alone for a few minutes. She watched from the hallway as Mark punched it. As he hit it, it went all around the room on the rod on the ceiling and came back in front of him. What a smile Mark had as he continued this anxiety-relieving activity! The next day, when he heard the doctor's footsteps, he asked the nurse for the "punching bag," and he went at it. He was communicating his feelings through play with both his illustration on the bag and his actions with the bag. Every day for the next 4 days, Mark performed the same activity prior to the doctor arriving. During this period, he was calmer, his vital signs remained stable, and he was in control. When Mark was finally discharged, he asked to take his "punching bag" home with him. He even asked the doctor to sign it, which he did. Play, the ultimate communication technique of children, was very effective in this case.

"doll play," and more technical medical play with the school-aged child. Older children may enjoy play activities on the computer such as participating in an online support group or sending email to the nurse. For the more sophisticated play of the adolescent, include more advanced computer activities such as creating a web page to tell their story and sharing it with others such as the nurse or other adolescents experiencing a similar problem. All of these play activities serve as a means of safe, acceptable communication between the child and the nurse.

Imaginary Friends

Imaginary friends are a form of play therapy that is often utilized by older preschoolers and school-age children. Their desire to communicate in the third person makes the use of an imaginary friend acceptable to them and an avenue from which they can communicate about themselves without acknowledging the connection. Imaginary friends "arrive" for a reason and, thus, should not be ignored

or criticized. Imaginary friends serve a purpose for children. Children talk to the "friend"; they allow their friend to talk for them, expressing how they feel, while maintaining their own inner self. Nurses and parents need to acknowledge the friend and allow this "friendship" to run its course. When the child no longer needs an imaginary friend, the friend will go away.

CONCLUSION

Communication with children is not defined by a script, by generalities, or by steadfast rules. Communication with children is dictated by each child's unique characteristics, including his or her age, cognitive development, language development, experiences, and the ability to express him- or herself through both verbal and nonverbal means. A child's ability to communicate changes and evolves over time. Nurses must be aware that communicating with a child involves appreciating the uniqueness of that child, having a general understanding of the physical and psychosocial development of children, having the patience to allow the child to express him- or herself using a variety of traditional and nontraditional methods, and being flexible. Two guiding principles are (1) no two children are alike, and (2) children are not miniature adults. To communicate with children effectively, the nurse must see the world through their eyes.

REFERENCES

1. Wong D. *Nursing Care of Infants and Children*. St. Louis: CV Mosby; 1999.

2. Chitty K. *Professional Nursing: Concepts and Challenges*. St. Louis: WB Saunders; 2001.

3. Deering C, Cody D. Communicating with children and adolescents. *American Journal of Nursing*. 2002;102(3):34-41.

4. Boggs K. Communicating with children. In: Arnold E, Boggs K, eds. *Interpersonal Relationships: Professional Communication Skills for Nurses*. 3rd ed. Philadelphia: WB Saunders; 1999.

5. Sydnor-Greenberg N, Dokken D. Communication in healthcare: thoughts on the child's perception. *Journal of Child and Family Nursing*. 2001;4(3):225-230.

6. Dossey B, Keegan L, Guzzetta C, Kolkmeier L. *Holistic Nursing: A Handbook for Practice*. Gaithersburg, Md: Aspen Publishing; 2001.

7. Color Kinetics Incorporated. *Consumer Products*. 10 Milk Street, Suite 1100, Boston, MA 02108. Accessed March 22, 2004 from:http://www.colorkinetics.com/products/consumer/details/index.htm?prd_id=69

8. DiGallo A. Drawing as a means of communication at the initial interview with children with cancer. *Journal of Child Psychotherapy*. 2001;27(2):197-210.

Exercises

1. Self-Assessment

Working with children is both exciting and challenging. Seeing the world through their eyes takes some imagination. It may help you recall your own childhood experiences with illness. Imagine a time when you were a child and you were ill, required surgery, or you were hospitalized. In your self-assessment notebook, communicate this experience either through a writing exercise (story, poem, narrative) or by drawing a picture depicting what that experience was like for you. Spend 5 to 10 minutes sharing those experiences with a confidant.

2. Responding to Situations

A. Suzy, an 11-year-old, is admitted to your unit for corrective surgery for scoliosis. You must complete preoperative teaching with her. Based on her age and cognitive level (she is age appropriate), what is the best communication technique to utilize with Suzy and why? Specifically, develop age- and cognitively appropriate teaching strategies to teach Suzy what she should expect.

B. Interpret the following (in writing) from the point of view of a toddler:

✳ "It will feel like a mosquito bite."

✳ "It is just a quick stick in your leg."

✳ "You are just going to have your cast cut off."

✳ "You sound like you are going to cough your head off."

✳ "I need to take some blood from you."

Now develop age-specific methods for communicating these ideas to toddlers using words or other appropriate methods.

✳ "It will feel like a mosquito bite."

✳ "It is just a quick stick in your leg."

✳ "You are just going to have your cast cut off."

✳ "You sound like you are going to cough your head off."

✳ "I need to take some blood from you."

Communicating With Cognitively Impaired Patients

Christine L. Williams, DNSc, RN, BC

OBJECTIVES

1. To differentiate between delirium and dementia
2. To describe nurse and client responses to cognitive impairment
3. To delineate therapeutic communication strategies for clients with cognitive impairment
4. To compare and contrast task-focused and emotion-focused communication
5. To adjust communication approaches to the severity of the client's cognitive impairment

INTRODUCTION

Because of the growing number of individuals living to old age worldwide, clients in many health care settings are older than age 65. Although cognitive impairment is not a normal condition in old age, it is much more common in the aged. Older adults who are hospitalized are at high risk for cognitive impairment during their hospital stays. Cognitive impairment may be a symptom of illness at the time of admission or it may develop as a result of anesthesia or other conditions such as dehydration. Most residents in long-term care experience some cognitive impairment as well. Whether a nurse provides care in the home, clinic, or other health care setting, he or she is likely to meet older adults and clients of all ages who are experiencing cognitive impairment.[1]

One type of cognitive impairment is *dementia*, which is caused by degenerative brain diseases, chronic alcoholism, human immunodeficiency virus (HIV), and other medical conditions.[2] Another type is *delirium*, which is caused by fever, electrolyte imbalance, sensory disturbances, or adverse reactions to drugs. Dementia and delirium differ in fundamental ways. Because the communication strategies nurses must implement with clients who are exhibiting dementia and delirium are somewhat different, they will be discussed separately.

DEMENTIA

Dementia is a gradual loss of cognitive ability that usually occurs during old age. Half of all older adults over the age of 85 have dementia.[3] It is never a normal or expected part of aging. It occurs with brain pathology and must be evaluated to determine if the dementia is reversible. The most common cause of dementia, Alzheimer's disease, is irreversible, but medications may slow the progression of the illness. Other causes of dementia include stroke and HIV.

The individual with dementia loses two or more cognitive abilities, such as memory impairment and apraxia (impaired ability to carry out motor activities in spite of having normal sensory abilities and understanding of the task). Aphasia, or deteriorating language, is another common cognitive loss. Aphasia results in difficulty verbally expressing thoughts and emotions, as well as difficulty in understanding verbal messages.[4] Cognitive losses gradually increase over a period of months or years. Although the individual remains alert, he or she eventually loses the ability to understand verbal communication as well. The result is a slower response to a question or command and frequent miscommunication.

NURSE AND CLIENT RESPONSES TO COGNITIVE IMPAIRMENT

Clients' emotional responses to cognitive loss will influence their overall mental health and ongoing relationships. As clients develop dementia, cognitive abilities decline at different rates. They retain many cognitive abilities, while other cognitive skills deteriorate. Clients who are painfully aware of their limitations may be reluctant to try to communicate. They may feel ashamed and withdraw from relationships or activities.[5]

Case Example

Mrs. Trescott, age 86, has lived a full and active life. She held positions of responsibility and enjoyed leadership status in her community. She recalls fond memories of winning her golf club championship several years in a row. Presently, she lives in a long-term care facility and has Alzheimer's disease. Although she is unable to care for herself, she speaks about the indignities of living in a sheltered environment. She is embarrassed about attending group exercise classes because the routines are well below her ability level. At the same time, she can be loud and disruptive in social activities and must be closely supervised.

Frustration, anger, and anxiety are common human responses for any individual who loses the ability to communicate verbally. When losses are gradual and relentless, such as in dementia, decreased self-esteem and depression are common and further interfere with the ability to communicate. With little hope for improvement and frequent awkward misunderstandings, it is not surprising that clients would wish to avoid communicating. Caregivers are also subject to the same frustration and anxiety when their attempts to communicate with the person who has cognitive limitations are unsuccessful. Mutual avoidance and withdrawal can be the result.[6,7] Many strategies are available for nurses to use to increase their chances of successful communication with these clients (Table 7-1). As you develop knowledge and skill you will more likely approach cognitively impaired clients with confidence rather than anxiety. Approaches to communication must be adapted not only to the person's ability to understand but to the purpose of the interaction. What is appropriate for assessment may be a barrier to communication that is designed to facilitate expression of concerns and feelings.

BALANCING THE NEED TO KNOW WITH THE CLIENT'S NEED FOR DIGNITY

During the nurse's evaluation of the client's cognitive and communication abilities, the client's deficits are exposed. This exposure is frequently stressful and embarrassing to the client. It is important for the nurse to be especially supportive and to convey respect for the worth and dignity of the person. Prepare clients in advance for questions that may be difficult to answer. Let clients know that it is okay if they do not know the answer. Some persons with dementia wonder aloud about the cause of their cognitive impairment and are self-critical. They may comment that they have become "stupid," "crazy," or they are "losing their mind." You can assure them that their memory problems do not have any relationship to such negative self-evaluations.

To provide safe and effective care, it is often necessary for the nurse to conduct an assessment of the client's cognitive ability. The Mini Mental State Examination (MMSE) is one test used to evaluate cognitive functioning in several areas including orientation, registration, attention, calculation, recall, and language.[4] The MMSE is used in assessing clients with cognitive impairment as well as those who are at risk for dementia, such as older adults or those with HIV or chronic substance abuse. The test can be introduced to the individual as a routine series of questions—some of which may be easy and others difficult to answer. The person with dementia will be unable to answer some and maybe all of the questions, and will commonly react with discomfort and dismay. Therefore, the test-taking situation is less threatening for the client when the nurse has established a trusting relationship and time is allowed to establish rapport before the test begins.

Table 7-1

GUIDELINES FOR COMMUNICATION WITH COGNITIVELY IMPAIRED PERSONS

Strategy	*Explanation*

Simplify your message
  Use common words and short sentences
  Ask one question at a time
	Aphasia limits the person's ability to understand complex verbal messages.

Accept the client's message	Persons with dementia may confuse the date or use one word and mean another. By avoiding correcting mistakes, the nurse demonstrates supportiveness.
Allow extra time If there is no response, try repeating the message or use different words and gestures	Cognitive impairment slows comprehension, wait for a response.
Break tasks down into simple steps Give instructions one step at a time	Cognitive impairment interferes with remembering multiple steps.
Avoid the use of pronouns Repeat names so that your message is clear	Cognitive impairment interferes with remembering the word or name to which the pronoun refers.
Use a calming approach	Conversation can be stressful. A soothing tone and an unhurried approach may prevent the client from feeling overwhelmed.
Take a break, try again later If you or the client becomes frustrated, try another approach at a later time	Miscommunication can be trying for both the nurse and the person with dementia. Maintaining a warm and supportive relationship is of utmost importance.

Clients should be advised to do their best in answering and should be assured that not knowing an answer does not necessarily mean that something is wrong. In fact, the individual only needs to obtain a score of 24 out of 30 possible answers to be classified as unimpaired. For an individual with less than an eighth-grade education, normal scores are two points lower. For example, if the obtained score is 18 and the individual has less than eight grades of education, the adjusted score is 20.[8] If a potential cognitive impairment is identified by a low score, the client should be referred to a psychiatrist, a neurologist, or a psychologist for further evaluation of cognitive deficits.

Since testing can be uncomfortable for persons with cognitive impairment, such questions should be reserved for special purposes, including evaluation of clinical progress and research. Quizzing clients and thus exposing their deficits whenever care is given is not helpful because it can harm self-esteem. Quizzing is quite different from a therapeutic strategy designed to stimulate cognitive activity. If the goal of the interaction is maintaining or regaining cognitive function, it is more helpful to involve clients in conversation about topics they choose or in activities they enjoy.

ENGAGING THE CLIENT IN COMMUNICATION

The goals of communication for persons with cognitive impairment include understanding the client's needs, sharing experiences, and engaging the client in his or her own care. Table 7-1 presents some general guidelines that will facilitate successful communication with clients with cognitive impairment.

Reality orientation is a strategy that involves providing information to persons with cognitive impairment to help them maintain contact with reality.[5] For example, the nurse uses reality orientation in the following statement: "Mr. Jeffrey, my name is Beverly Tomez and I am your nurse. Today is Wednesday, January 23rd, and you are in the hospital." This statement is intended to reduce anxiety by reinforcing orientation to time and place. Although this strategy is not harmful when used occasionally, it has limited usefulness for interacting with the person with dementia.[2] Many people with dementia become embarrassed or frustrated when they realize that they have forgotten the date or where they are. Further, they are likely to forget the information in a few minutes; therefore, reminding them, particularly over and over again, is not helpful. Displaying a clock and calendar where they can be easily seen is more useful (and less threatening) since the information is available when the person needs it.

Facilitating Trust

Establishing trust with a person with dementia is a challenging but not impossible task. Once a trusting relationship is established, the goals of care are much easier to obtain. The person with dementia will remember that you are trustworthy, although he or she may not remember all of the details of the experience that led to the feeling of trust.

The short-term effect of the dishonesty in the case example is that the resident may get onto the elevator. Later, the person with dementia may become disruptive and uncooperative and will be unlikely to trust in what the nursing assistant tells her. A better approach would be to encourage a trusted family member or consistent caregiver to be present at the time of the appointment, to allow extra time to accompany the resident, and to ensure that the caregiver uses a calming approach. If the resident becomes agitated upon leaving the unit, this is an

---

Case Example

You are a nurse in a long-term care facility and a resident has an appointment with a specialist in a location off the unit. The nursing assistant is trying to persuade the resident to accompany her to the appointment, and the resident is anxious and reluctant to get onto the elevator. Hoping to gain the resident's cooperation, the nursing assistant tells the resident that her son is waiting and she must get into the elevator if she wants to see him. What would you do?

---

issue that can be discussed with the family and interdisciplinary team. It may be possible for a small dose of an as-needed medication for anxiety to be given in advance of the appointment or perhaps the care provider can come to the unit for a meeting.

Avoid talking about the person with cognitive impairment in his or her presence. Address the client directly instead of speaking to a nearby family member or coworker. Use the client's formal name and ask what he or she would like to be called. Avoid endearments such as "Dear" or "Mamma," which imply a social relationship rather than a professional one. Remember, cognitively impaired clients are adults, although some of their behavior may seem child-like.

Task-Focused Communication

When nurses request specific information from clients (eg, "Are you in pain?") or give directions (eg, "Take this medicine"), they are using task-focused communication. The following approaches are guidelines for this type of interaction.

Because the individual may have difficulty understanding complex messages, keep your messages simple and direct. Present one idea at a time. Ask for what you want rather than what you do not want. For example, it is easier for persons with dementia to understand a statement, such as "Hold the glass with both hands," than it is for them to understand a negatively worded command, such as "Careful, don't spill your drink!"

Complex questions are also unlikely to produce a useful response. Asking two questions at once is confusing even to the person without cognitive impairment. Asking "why" requires analysis of reasons for behavior and sounds like a challenge or confrontation. For example, "Why did you put your coat on?

It's hot outside!" This question is unlikely to produce a positive response. Instead, it would be better to preserve the person's sense of dignity with a supportive response: "Let me help you put your coat away. It is very hot out today. I don't think you will need it."

Do not overburden persons with cognitive impairment with unnecessary information. In orienting them to a new living environment, for example, it may be more appropriate to include essential information about their immediate surroundings at first (such as where the bathroom is and how they can call for help) rather than an orientation to the entire unit. Allow for slower processing of information by giving additional time for questions.

In order to gain your clients' cooperation, avoid increasing their anxiety. A statement such as "If you can't stay in bed, I will have to put the side rails up!" is not likely to be of any help. Clients may not remember the details of such a threat a few minutes later, but they will feel less secure in their new surroundings. When the nurse remembers to plan care to accommodate persons with cognitive deficits, less frustration will occur.

By giving simple choices and allowing some flexibility, the nurse empowers clients to participate in their care. For example, the nurse asks, "Would you like to wash your face?" (while handing the washcloth to the client), thereby encouraging the person to choose to participate rather than become the passive recipient of care.

Arguing with someone who is cognitively impaired is unlikely to gain cooperation and will only escalate frustration and agitation. For example, Mrs. Silva shouts at the nursing assistant, "You stole my teeth!" Rather than defending herself and arguing that Mrs. Silva misplaced her own dentures, the nursing assistant wisely responds, "Let me help you find your dentures, Mrs. Silva."

Emotion-Focused Communication

Contrary to popular belief, clients with dementia can form therapeutic relationships with their nurses. Despite memory deficits, these clients have the same emotional needs as any other person including the need for relationships with others. In a study of nursing home residents with advanced dementia, nurses visited three times weekly over a period of 16 weeks.[5] During that time, residents remembered that they had a relationship with the nurses and frequently brought up what was discussed at previous sessions, although they may not have remembered the nurses' names. They also chose to discuss their emotions and concerns. Some of the topics included death, loneliness, isolation, and relationships with family members. It was not unusual for residents to discuss their feelings about the nurse (eg, "I missed you!").

Care providers frequently assume that because cognitively impaired persons have difficulty finding the words to express ideas, they have lost their individuality, their humanity, and, in some cases, their entire "self." This sense of who they are in fact persists over the course of the dementing illness.[7] Recognition of the person as a person is necessary to maintain quality of life.

Most communication is nonverbal, therefore, nurses can understand much about a person by being observant. Feelings are expressed with facial expressions, posture, tone of voice, and gestures. It is not necessary for clients to tell us in words that they are frightened or angry. Anxiety can be communicated with overall body tension or facial expressions such as worry lines, wide eyes, or eyes that seem to scan the environment for a threat. Anger may be portrayed by banging the hand on an object, yelling, or a tightly held fist. Slumped posture or the chin propped up with a hand may indicate discouragement or depression. Many persons with dementia who have limited speech become agitated and restless when they are experiencing strong emotions. When agitation occurs, assume that the person is distressed and begin searching for the cause. Look for situational cues. What happened just before the person became agitated? Ask for validation of what you perceive (eg, "You seem frightened.").

If the client has limited speech, assume that he or she hears and understands at least some of what is being communicated. Respect for the dignity of the person is conveyed in many subtle ways. If you relax and sit down before beginning a conversation, you convey "I have time for you." It may only be a few minutes, but you can give the individual your full attention for whatever time you have. The strategies listed in Table 7-2 can be used to guide the nurse in emotion-focused conversations with clients who are cognitively impaired.[6]

It is especially important to provide the healing presence of a nurse during important life changes and

---

Table 7-2

GUIDELINES FOR EMOTION-FOCUSED COMMUNICATION

Strategy	Explanation
Making time	Sitting with the client, making eye contact, and using touch provides the atmosphere for emotion-focused conversation.
Being receptive	Acknowledging concerns and emotions encourages expression.
Broad openings	Beginning with general questions and statements encourages clients to choose what to talk about.
Speaking as equals	Relating to clients as persons with something to offer in the relationship facilitates trust.
Establishing commonalities	Sharing experiences can be a way of developing and deepening the relationship between nurse and client.
Maintaining the conversation	Following up on important concerns and emotions facilitates the flow of conversation.

---

times of crisis. We can assume that people with dementia will have emotional responses to major events in their lives just as any other person would. If a long-time resident of an assisted living facility has to be moved to the nursing home due to increasing frailty, the nurse can assume that the resident will experience anxiety and loss, and will be at risk for agitation and depression. In anticipation, the nurse needs to arrange opportunities for support. Spending time with the person with dementia will provide the opportunity to observe and listen for the emotions expressed with or without words. Although the words in a conversation may be difficult to follow, emotions can be understood nonverbally, as discussed.

Allowing and even encouraging expression of negative emotions such as anger and grief can be therapeutic. Persons with dementia need to know that someone hears their distress and will be with them and respond with empathy. Commonly, unpleasant emotions are dismissed by distracting cognitively impaired persons with pleasant thoughts and activities. It is important to give them the opportunity to express their feelings and receive support. These periods of emotional expression can be balanced with pleasant activities as well. It is not therapeutic to deny painful feelings nor is it helpful to dwell on them to the exclusion of enjoying other activities.

Facilitating discussion of sensitive topics is important, but clients' limitations need to be considered as well. Clients who are cognitively intact remember painful events under discussion (such as the death of a loved one) and remember prior discussions of the event. Persons with cognitive impairment may react to discussion of painful events as if they are hearing about it for the first time. Being therapeutic involves adjusting your approach to this reality. The following case example illustrates this point.

In a study of communication strategies used by nurses, several strategies were identified as helpful in encouraging the expression of feelings in individuals with dementia.[6] Using *broad openings* is one strategy. A question as simple as "How are you?" encourages discussion and allows the person to respond in whatever way he or she can to communicate concerns. It does not limit the client to a "yes" or "no" answer, as "Are you upset?" would.

Case Example

An 89-year-old woman is wandering on the dementia unit and calling out for her husband, who died more than 10 years ago. She appears sad and anxious and is becoming agitated. One response might be to tell her that her husband is working and he will be home later that day. This explanation may even seem to calm her for the moment; however, a feeling of uncertainty and mistrust may result when the promised reunion does not occur.

Another approach to this situation is brutal honesty. Telling her that her husband passed away and that she now lives in a nursing home rather than with her husband may result in tearfulness and distress. With this response, the tears may be quieted with comforting, but the individual with memory loss may be calling out for her husband again a few minutes later.

Instead, it is possible to respond supportively without doing harm. If she misses her husband she may benefit by reminiscing about him. Ask her to tell you about her husband and about her life with him. This approach allows her to meet a need to remember her husband without cutting off discussion of this sensitive subject.

Another successful strategy is referred to as *speaking as equals.* This means creating a climate of respect in which the interviewer views the client as someone to learn from and someone of equal value in the relationship. *Establishing commonalities* is another helpful strategy that means sharing perceptions or interests. The following case example illustrates sharing perceptions.

Sharing of self involves the nurse offering his or her feelings or thoughts in the conversation with the person with dementia. Positive feelings are expressed verbally or nonverbally with touch. When nurses share their feelings, they reinforce the idea that a valued relationship exists between two people.

Maintaining the conversation is a strategy that encompasses efforts to continue the interaction despite unclear verbalizations. Nurses listen for reoccurring themes in conversation and summarize what they hear in order to help persons with dementia express concerns and emotions. By verbalizing themes and asking clients for validation, the nurse checks for accuracy of understanding. "You have been talking about all the things you miss about your home in Chicago. Are you feeling sad today?" Nurses

Case Example

Mrs. Jackson, a 90-year-old resident of a dementia unit in a nursing home, has limited speech. The nurse spent a few minutes with Mrs. Jackson after another resident had become extremely agitated in the dining area and was led away. Mrs. Jackson remarked, "It's crazy in this place!" The nurse shares her perception that "it is very confusing here this morning."

use nonverbal and verbal encouragers (head nodding and "uh-huh") to assist clients to elaborate.

Nurses may be uncomfortable and may even avoid interaction when they do not understand persons with dementia. Those with cognitive losses and accompanying communication deficits may avoid confronting their losses and withdraw as well. The nurse who is skilled in communicating can prevent clients' isolation and thus play an important role in enhancing quality of life for persons with dementia.

Adjusting Communication to the Stage of Dementia

As clients move into the later stages of a dementing illness, communication strategies must be adapted to their declining language abilities. Decline in the number of words a client uses and in the relevance of responses is common. For some clients, verbalizations are long and repetitive and lack relevance to a topic. *Mutism* gradually occurs for others. This means speaking may become less and less frequent until verbal communication ceases. In the final stages of dementia, the individual seems unaware of his or her surroundings.[9]

As verbal abilities decline, the client must put forth greater and greater effort to communicate. Adjust the amount of time you expect the client to engage in conversation accordingly. Someone with minimal impairment may enjoy 30 minutes of conversation, while the individual with more severe impairment may only tolerate 15 minutes. Take your cues from the client. With regular opportunities to converse, most clients can increase the amount of time spent in conversation with a trusted caregiver.

During the later stages of dementia, it is still important to remember that the client may understand more than you realize. Continue to narrate what you do in a calming voice. Address the client by name and use gentle touch on an arm or shoulder to focus his or her attention. Use supportive facial expressions, such as smiling and eye contact. Use gestures to reinforce verbal messages. Assume the client can understand and ask for his or her cooperation as you provide care. Many caregivers can relate experiences in which persons with advanced dementia surprised them with an action or statement that indicated much more awareness than expected. Knowing that you have communicated successfully with someone who is difficult to reach is a very rewarding experience.[10]

DELIRIUM

Delirium is another common condition that is characterized by cognitive impairment, disturbance of consciousness, and communication problems. It occurs over a short period of time (hours or days) and is considered a medical emergency. The person's level of consciousness may change from alert to lethargic. A few hours later, he or she may be difficult to arouse or hyperalert. Inattentiveness and disorganized thinking are also common.[4,11]

Delirium is caused by an underlying physical problem, such as infection or toxic reaction to a medication.[12] Rapid identification of the underlying problem is critical so that corrective action can be taken. To provide a feeling of safety for the client, the nurse should use a calming approach both verbally and nonverbally, thus limiting the anxiety that the client will inevitably experience in such a situation. Unhurried actions and a soothing tone of voice will contribute to the overall calming effect of the nurse's behavior. The guidelines for communication with cognitively impaired persons identified in Table 7-1 are also appropriate to use with the person experiencing delirium.

A professional nurse should closely monitor such a client to prevent harm from agitated behavior and a rapidly changing condition. Speak to the client even though you may not be sure you are heard and understood. Clients who have experienced delirium may tell you that they remember the nurse as a source of comfort and reassurance.

Disorganized thinking will limit the amount of information clients can comprehend. Remind clients of who you are and what they can expect to reduce anxiety caused by the unfamiliar situation. For example, "Mr. Brown, I am your nurse Jeffrey Levine, you are in the hospital, and I will be taking care of you today." As a client's condition changes, be prepared to alter your verbal approach. Use moments of increased alertness as opportunities to interact and reinforce orienting information.

Explain what you are doing but use simple terms and repeat your message often. Encourage family members to sit with the client and provide touch and a calming presence. It is much better to use close observation by a person to maintain safety than it is to use restraints.[13] Help the client to explore tubes and lines with you as you guide his or her hands and briefly explain what he or she is touching. Move tubes and lines away from the client's field of vision to reduce the chance that he or she will pull at them during periods of clouded consciousness.

The methods described in this chapter for emotion-focused communication with persons with dementia are of limited use for persons with delirium. The delirious client needs to trust that he or she is safe and is being cared for, while every effort is made to identify and reverse the underlying problem that is causing the delirium. Consistent caregivers, gentle touch, patience, and a soothing tone of voice contribute to building trust.

CONCLUSION

Communicating with clients who are cognitively impaired is challenging. Cognitively impaired clients may resist care because they are frightened or depressed. It is important to develop trust and to avoid the use of force in providing care. The use of mechanical restraints has been shown to cause significant harm emotionally and physically, and the consequences may persist long after the episode has ended.[13] If combative behavior or resistance to care does occur, ask for help from the interdisciplinary team. A consult from a psychiatrist will be necessary to determine the appropriate medication for severe psychiatric symptoms and combativeness. Develop a consistent approach so that nurses on every shift will respond to these clients consistently.

REFERENCES

1. Hendrix-Bedalow PM. Alzheimer's dementia: coping with communication decline. *Journal of Gerontological Nursing.* 2000;26(8):20-24.
2. Small GW, Rabins PV, Barry PP, et al. Diagnosis and treatment of Alzheimer's disease and related disorders: consensus

statement of the American Association for Geriatric Psychiatry, the Alzheimer's Association, and the American Geriatrics Society. *JAMA.* 1997;278:1363-1371.

3. Beck CK, Shue VM. Interventions for treating disruptive behavior in demented elderly people. *Nursing Clinics of North America.* 1994;29(1):143-155.

4. American Psychiatric Association. *Diagnostic and Statistical Manual of Mental Disorders.* 4th ed. Washington DC: American Psychiatric Association; 2000.

5. Williams C, Tappen R. Can we create a therapeutic relationship with nursing home residents in the later stages of Alzheimer's disease? *Journal of Psychosocial Nursing and Mental Health Services.* 1999;37(3):1-8.

6. Tappen R, Williams-Burgess C, Edelstein J, Touhy T, Fishman S. Communicating with individuals with Alzheimer's disease: examination of recommended strategies. *Archives of Psychiatric Nursing.* 1997;11(5):249-256.

7. Tappen R., Williams C, Fishman S, Touhy T. Persistence of self in advanced Alzheimer's disease. *Image: The Journal for Nursing Scholarship.* 1999;31(2):121-125.

8. O'Connor DW, Pollitt PA, Treasure FP, Brook CP, Reiss BB. The influence of education, social class and sex on Mini-Mental State scores. *Psychological Medicine.* 1989;19:771-776.

9. Olga V, Emery B. Language impairment in dementia of the Alzheimer's type: a hierarchical decline? *International Journal of Psychiatry in Medicine.* 2000;30(2):145-164.

10. Edberg AK, Nordmark Sandgren A, Hallberg, IR. Initiating and terminating verbal interaction between nurses and severely demented patients regarded as vocally disruptive. *Journal of Psychiatric and Mental Health Nursing.* 1995;2:159-167.

11. Henry M. Descending into delirium. *American Journal of Nursing.* 2002;102(3):49-56.

12. Spar JE, LaRue A. *Concise Guide to Geriatric Psychiatry.* 3rd ed. Washington DC: American Psychiatric Association; 2002.

13. Rogers PD, Bocchino NL. Restraint-free care: is it possible? *American Journal of Nursing.* 1999;99(10):27-34.

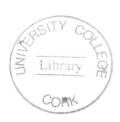

EXERCISES

1. Self-Assessment

Working with aging adults can be both challenging and rewarding. Use these exercises to help you develop self-understanding about caring for older clients.

A. List 10 words that come to mind when you picture someone who is "old."

1.
2.
3.
4.
5.
6.
7.
8.
9.
10.

Are these words mostly positive or negative? As a result of this exercise, what have you learned about your beliefs about aging?

B. What do you think it means to be "healthy" in old age?

C. Feeling empathy for someone who is in late life can be difficult when our experiences seem so different. It may help to do the following exercise. Picture yourself at age 85.

✳ What do you look like?

✳ Where are you living?

✳ With whom do you enjoy spending time?

✳ What do you enjoy doing?

✳ What is most important to you?

✳ What are your greatest joys?

✳ What brings you sadness?

✳ What do you see as your major health problem?

Discussion

Write a brief summary of what you think it might be like to be old. If you were old, what would you like your nurse to do or say?

2. Responding to Situations

Below are situations in which you might find yourself as you interact with clients with cognitive impairments in the clinical setting. These situations are posed to help you better understand the process of therapeutic interaction.

A. Your client, Mr. Schneider, is 90 years old and admitted to the hospital from the nursing home with severe health problems including severe confusion. When you visit him in his room to conduct an initial assessment, you note that he screams whenever you touch him.

* ✳ What do you think Mr. Schneider feels in this situation?

* ✳ What might you feel in this situation?

* ✳ What could you say and or do that might be helpful for Mr. Schneider?

B. Mrs. Jacobs, age 87, was admitted to the hospital for repair of a fractured hip. She fell at home, where she lives with her family. You are the evening nurse assigned to her care. You notice that she seems confused although this was not mentioned in the shift report. She is crying but does answer your questions about pain.

* ✳ What might you be feeling in this situation?

* ✳ What would be a good outcome in this situation?

* ✳ Is there really anything that you can do that will help?

Discussion

In your self-assessment notebook, summarize what you have learned in doing this exercise. What kinds of feelings do you experience in caring for older persons with cognitive impairments? How do you handle those feelings? What would you like to change about the way you approach elders with cognitive impairment?

Communicating With Critically Ill, Mechanically Ventilated Clients

Nancy E. Villanueva, PhD, ARNP, BC, CNRN

OBJECTIVES

1. To examine the barriers to communication that exist when caring for mechanically ventilated clients
2. To discuss the importance of communication from the client's perspective
3. To describe methods or techniques that may assist the nurse to communicate with mechanically ventilated clients

INTRODUCTION

As discussed throughout this book, effective communication is essential to the relationship between the nurse and client. The ability to communicate is often taken for granted, and it is not appreciated until the nurse finds him- or herself in a situation in which the traditional means of communication are not possible. Nurses who practice in an intensive care unit provide care to clients who are unable to communicate verbally or nonverbally. For the client who is mechanically ventilated without cognitive impairment, the ability to speak is lost, but nonverbal communication remains possible. In contrast, the client who has a cognitive impairment (eg, unconsciousness) and is mechanically ventilated has lost both verbal and nonverbal communication.

VOICELESSNESS

Voicelessness has been identified as the inability to speak resulting from respiratory tract intubation and/or mental status changes (permanent or transient).[1] Clients who have experienced voicelessness describe feelings of insecurity, frustration, anxiety/fear, anger, agony, and panic.[2-4] Asking a question or expressing a need is a challenge for the intubated client. Trying to get the nurse to understand what the client is asking for can be an exhausting and frustrating experience. This sense of frustration can be seen in one client's statement: "I can remember getting cross with everybody, getting cross with... my husband, my sister, my mum and dad because they couldn't understand what I was to say to them."[4] In one study, clients were interviewed about their experiences with communication while intubated. Thirteen of the 22 clients interviewed felt that the registered nurse caring for them was able to understand their needs and wishes.[5]

Other frustrations arise from insufficient explanations and inadequate understanding of conversations with caregivers. Explanations related to the client's care and treatments are not clearly understood and the client is unable to communicate the need for additional information and clarification. Also frustrating is the inability of the nurse to interpret the client's nonverbal cues, which results in misunder-standing of the client's request or continued attempts to communicate.[1,2,4,6]

BARRIERS TO COMMUNICATION WITH THE CRITICALLY ILL CLIENT

The intensive care unit presents many barriers to effective nurse-client communication. Bassett[2] placed the various barriers in two categories: *mechanical* and *psychological.* Included in the mechanical category is the client's inability to speak or communicate. Factors that influence this category include the client's medical condition, the administration of sedating and neuromuscular blocking agents (NMBAs), presence of an artificial airway, and the noise generated by the various pieces of equipment in the intensive care unit.

Communication is an active process that requires energy. The client who is critically ill may not have the energy necessary to communicate or may only have a limited reserve that becomes depleted with repeated attempts to communicate. In an interview, one client explained that she did not want to make an effort to communicate but wanted to be understood with as few gestures as possible.[4]

The medications utilized also influence the abili-ty to communicate. NMBAs are frequently employed in the care of critically ill clients. These agents paralyze the skeletal muscles and render individuals unable to move, breathe, or even open their eyes. However, the medication does not alter consciousness and is not analgesic, sedative, or amnestic in nature. For these clients, verbal and nonverbal communication is lost. The administra-tion of sedating agents to mechanically ventilated clients also affects their ability to communicate by altering their mental status.[7]

FACTORS INFLUENCING NURSE-CLIENT COMMUNICATION

There are factors that may both limit and facilitate communication with intubated clients depending on the situation. Some of the factors identified by criti-cal care nurses that limit their ability to communicate include[1,7-9]:
* The acuity of the client
* The individual nurse's client assignment

* Inability to speak the client's language
* Difficulty reading the client's lips
* Inability of the client to write and/or read
* Continuity of client assignments
* Experience level of the nurse
* Presence of family and/or significant others
* Insufficient training in communication skills

Additional factors were identified when the client was comatose or unresponsive due to NMBAs. These factors included self-consciousness on the part of the nurse, lack of privacy, and the circumstances sur-rounding the injury. The nurses who were inter-viewed described feeling self-conscious talking to a client who was unable to talk back or use nonverbal methods. The majority of communication with clients consisted of informing them of upcoming pro-cedures or activities. Rarely were nonprocedural top-ics discussed.[7]

The experience level of the nurse is a factor that can also inhibit communication. A grounded theory study by Villanueva[7] explored the experiences of critical care nurses caring for clients who were com-atose due to a traumatic head injury or receiving an NMBA. As novices, the nurses described themselves as being task-oriented, overwhelmed, and intimidat-ed. Their focus was on managing the complex equip-ment and required nursing responsibilities. It was not until novices achieved a comfort level with the tech-nical aspects of the role that they were able to focus on talking to clients. Clients' acuity was also a factor in inhibited communication, even for experienced nurses. The higher the clients' acuity, the greater the intensity required for monitoring physiological and neurological status, maintaining the complex equip-ment, and performing the numerous nursing respon-sibilities. As a result, the nurses talked less to their clients, and when they did talk, the conversation was limited to information about upcoming procedures or activities.

Factors that have been found to facilitate commu-nication with the client include the client's ability to interact using nonverbal techniques and knowing about the client as a person. The presence of family and/or significant others allows the nurse to come to know the client as a person. Through interactions with the family, the nurse is able to learn about the client and his or her life. This information allows the nurse to provide individualized communication when talking to the client. An example of this can be seen in the following situation: The nurse knows from the family that the client is an avid sports fan, and when talking to the client, the nurse will include information related to recent sports events (eg, Sunday football games and scores).[7,8] The presence of family can also assist in helping the nurse understand the client's nonverbal communication. Family members are familiar with the client's gestures, facial expressions, and frequently are able to more easily interpret what the client is trying to communicate. Also, the family may be able to read the client's lips more clearly than the nurse.[1]

In two grounded theory studies, experienced intensive care nurses identified "maintaining continuity in client assignments" as a factor that promotes communication with clients. Having continuity in assignments allowed the nurses to come to know the client's nonverbal behaviors, facial expressions, and moods. Having this knowledge allowed them to be able to interpret what the client was trying to say more effectively and accurately.[7,10]

AUGMENTATIVE COMMUNICATION METHODS

A variety of communication tools can be utilized with the intubated client. The tools that are currently available do have client requirements in order for them to be effective. Clearly, for any tool the client must be awake, alert, and have effective cognitive function. Other requirements are dependent on the tool selected.

Tools range from simple to complex devices. Tools that are frequently used include writing pads, Magic Slate (Vic Enterprises, Tacoma, Wash), alphabet cards, and picture boards. All of these tools require the client to have sufficient energy, writing or pointing ability, vision, and concentration to use the tool. Keep in mind the intubated client has restricted head movement due to the endotracheal tube and ventilator tubing. This restriction may limit the use of some communication tools. The need for corrective lenses must also be addressed in order for the client to be able to see the tool being used.[8,11]

Another factor that must be taken into account when considering these tools is the client's ability to move an arm to point or ability to hold a pencil. Invasive monitoring lines, immobilization, or paralysis may restrict movement.[11]

In one study, a Magic Slate was used in an attempt to improve communication for clients with tracheostomies. Fifteen clients were asked to evaluate the effectiveness of the slate as a communication tool. Results showed that 73% of the clients felt the tool appropriate for their condition, 86% felt it facilitated communication with the health care team, and the slate was accepted by 96% of the clients.[12]

An alphabet card and/or a picture board can be used for clients who do not possess the ability to write or point. The picture board can also be used when the nurse does not speak the client's language. Alphabet cards are available commercially or may be written out by the nursing staff. The size is usually 8 x 12" and the letters are arranged in rows. To use the card, the nurse points to a line and asks the client if the word begins with a letter on that line. If the letter is not on that line, the nurse points to the next line and asks the same question. Once the correct line is determined, the nurse points to each letter in the line. The client can indicate that the nurse has pointed to the correct letter by nodding his or her head or, if unable to move the head, by blinking his or her eyes. Spelling out a word using this technique is time-consuming and can be frustrating for the client as well as the nurse. If the client has the ability to point to the letters, time and frustration can be reduced.

Having an alphabet card was described by one client as a security blanket. Communicating without the card was very frustrating and the client feared the card would get lost or misplaced. It was important to keep the card within the client's field of vision at all times.[13]

Picture boards contain icons that depict a variety of basic needs to which the client points to express his or her needs to the nurse. Icons represent pain, hot and cold, thirst, and bedpan. Improvement in client-nurse communication was demonstrated in a study that utilized a picture board for intubated clients following cardiothoracic surgery.[8]

There are a variety of electronic voice output communication aids (VOCAs) that combine icons or pictures with prerecorded voice messages or synthesized speech. These devices are available through speech language departments and require a consult for a speech pathologist to assess the client's ability to use the device, then to provide the necessary instruction on use of the device. The devices may have a touch-sensitive screen in which the client touches the icon that represents what he or she is trying to communicate. Touch-sensitive keyboards are also utilized. Examples of preprogrammed messages include "I am having pain," "What time is it?" and "I am thirsty." Preoperative preparation allows the client to record messages using his or her own voice. In addition to the standard messages, the client can add personalized ones. The devices are mounted on an arm attached to the client's bedside. Having it positioned on the arm allows for the device to be moved into the best position for the client to access it.[8,14]

The Children's Hospital in Boston has developed a model of alternative communication interventions for clients who will remain intubated following surgery. In this model, the client and family work with the speech pathologist preoperatively to provide them with communication tools for use after surgery. If outpatient preoperative instruction is not possible, the instruction is provided in the operating room before the client receives sedation. Following surgery, the speech pathologist is contacted once the client is alert and able to use the communication tools. This contact is usually made once the client is in the intensive care unit. The speech language pathologist reassesses the client's alertness and motor and sensory skills to determine if any modifications need to be made to the previously selected communication aids. Clients who have participated in this model reported that they did not feel exhausted while attempting to communicate, isolated, or afraid because of communication problems.[14]

For clients with tracheostomies who meet the necessary criteria, a one-way Passy-Muir (Ohio State University Medical Center, Columbus, Ohio) speaking valve is available. The one-way valve directs the exhaled air around the tracheostomy tube, through the vocal cords, and into the oral and nasal cavities, allowing the client to speak. A consult with a speech language pathologist is required for client evaluation to determine readiness for use of the tube. Absolute contraindications include foam-cuffed tracheostomy tubes, inflated tracheostomy cuffs, laryngectomies, sleep, or coma. Apraxia, oral motor weakness, or dysarthria are conditions that exclude the client as a candidate. Respiratory muscle strength, secretions, and oxygenation must also be taken into consideration. The

length of time the valve is used increases as the client develops tolerance to the device. While the valve is in use, the nurse monitors the client's vital signs, oxygen saturation, work of breathing, and respiratory rate. The nurse collaborates with the respiratory therapist, who must adjust the ventilator settings to compensate for volume losses, F_1O_2, and positive end-expiratory pressure (PEEP). In addition to providing the ability to speak, the valve was found to improve swallowing skills, decrease secretions, and reestablish a sense of smell.[15,16]

IMPLICATIONS FOR NURSING PRACTICE

The importance of communication between nurses and mechanically ventilated clients has been well established along with the difficulties encountered when attempting to communicate. Nurses need to recognize the impact that voicelessness has on clients. By putting him- or herself in the client's place, the nurse is able to experience being voiceless.

Nurses must also recognize that gestures, facial expressions, body language, and space all affect meaning. In addition, the tone of voice, pitch, and cadence influence the interpretation of a statement.[17,18] Positioning of the client to allow him or her to see the nurse during communication attempts may facilitate the success of the interaction. However, the ability to position clients is dependent upon the physiological status, monitoring devices, and intravenous tubings.

Two strategies that may be utilized to determine if the nurse correctly understands what the client is attempting to communicate are (1) looking at the client's expression for evidence of relief or recognition, and (2) repeating back to the client what the nurse understands the client to be communicating. The client will indicate by a pre-established yes/no response if the message was correctly interpreted.[19]

When obtaining the client's history, it is important to ascertain if he or she wears glasses (reading or distance) or has problems hearing. Glasses may need to be modified to accommodate the client's condition. Take, for example, the client who has excessive facial swelling or a head dressing. In both of these situations, the arms of the frames will not fit. The arms can be removed and the glasses worn as spectacles. If the client has problems with hearing, is one ear better than the other? Or is a hearing aid used? If there is a hearing aid, it needs to be available for the client to use. The family should be asked to bring it in from home. If the client is unable to wear the hearing aid, it may be helpful to consult a speech/language pathologist to determine the availability of an auditory trainer/amplifier to assist the client.[14]

Whenever possible, communication tools should be a standard part of preoperative education for clients who will be mechanically ventilated after surgery. The client has the opportunity to practice using the selected tool prior to surgery. This provides a way for the client to communicate and decreases the feelings of insecurity, frustration, anxiety/fear, anger, agony, and panic that have been described by clients experiencing voicelessness.

In situations in which preoperative instruction is not possible, the nurse may select the communication tool best suited for the client. Nurses may consult and collaborate with speech/language pathologists for their suggestions regarding the most appropriate tool for the client. The use of communication tools requires nurses to become knowledgeable and comfortable working with these devices.

CONCLUSION

Communicating with the individual who is critically ill presents unique challenges for the nurse. Nurses must recognize the importance that communication represents for the client. The need to provide a way to achieve this communication should be given high priority. However, at times, the acuity of the client's physiological status requires the nurse's complete focus, and communication is limited to only the essential or technical aspects at that time. The voicelessness that accompanies mechanical ventilation is a common type of communication barrier requiring knowledge and skill to overcome. An experienced, competent nurse is better able to provide physical care while maintaining a focus on the client as a person. Advance planning when possible and augmentative communication devices can facilitate the client's ability to communicate and facilitate development and maintenance of a relationship with the mechanically ventilated client.

REFERENCES

1. Happ MB. Interpretation of nonvocal behavior and the meaning of voicelessness in critical care. *Social Science & Medicine.* 2000;50:1247-1255.

2. Bassett CC. Communication with the critically ill. *Care of the Critically Ill.* 1993;9(5):216-219.

3. Bergbom-Engberg I, Haljamae H. Assessment of clients' experience of discomforts during respirator therapy. *Critical Care Medicine.* 1989;17(10):1068-1072.

4. Todres L, Fulbrook P, Albarran J. On the receiving end: a hermeneutic-phenomenological analysis of a client's struggle to cope while going through intensive care. *Nursing in Critical Care.* 2000;5(6):277-287.

5. Wojnicki-Johansson G. Communication between nurse and client during ventilator treatment: client reports and RN evaluations. *Intensive & Critical Care Nursing.* 2001;17(1):29-39.

6. Connolly MA, Shekleton ME. Communicating with ventilator dependent clients. *Dimensions of Critical Care Nursing.* 1991;10(2):115-122.

7. Villanueva N. *Experiences of Critical Care Nurses Caring for Clients in Traumatic Coma or Pharmacological Paralysis.* Dissertation. Miami, Fla: University of Miami; 1997.

8. Happ MB. Communicating with mechanically ventilated clients: state of the science. *AACN Clinical Issues.* 2001;12(2):247-258.

9. Leathart AJ. Communication and socialization (1): an exploratory study and explanation for nurse-client communication in an ITU. *Intensive & Critical Care Nursing.* 1994;10:93-104.

10. Adler DC. *The Experience and Caring Needs of Critically Ill Mechanically Ventilated Clients.* Dissertation. Philadelphia: University of Pennsylvania; 1997.

11. Jablonski-Seeger RA. The experience of being mechanically ventilated. *Qualitative Health Research.* 1994;4:186-207.

12. Melles AM, Zago MMF. The magic blackboard in the promotion of written communication by tracheostomized clients. *Revista Latino-Americana de Enfermagem.* 2001;9(1):73-79.

13. Villaire M. ICU—from the client's point of view. *Critical Care Nurse.* 1995;Feb:81-87.

14. Costello JM. AAC intervention in the intensive care unit: the Children's Hospital Boston Model. *Augmentative and Alternative Communication.* 2000;16(3):137-153.

15. Kaut K, Turcott JC, Lavery M. Passy-Muir speaking valve. *Dimensions of Critical Care Nursing.* 1996;15(6):298-306.

16. Passy V, Baydur A, Prentice W, Darnell-Neal R. Passy-Muir tracheostomy speaking valve on ventilator-dependent clients. *Laryngoscope.* 1993;103:653-658.

17. Alibali MW, Heath DC, Myers HJ. Effects of visibility between speaker and listener on gesture production: some gestures are meant to be seen. *Journal of Memory and Language.* 2001;44(2):169-188.

18. Dreger V. Communication: an important assessment and teaching tool. *Insight.* 2001;26(2):57-60.

19. Hemsley B, Sigafoos J, Balandin S, et al. Nursing the client with severe communication impairment. *Journal of Advanced Nursing.* 2001;35(6):827-835.

EXERCISES

1. Self-Assessment

Working with critically ill adults can be both frightening and exciting. Caring for someone who is so dependent on you is a tremendous responsibility. Use these exercises to help you prepare for caring for clients who are critically ill and voiceless.

A.   What words come to mind when you picture yourself as a critical care or emergency room nurse? List them now:

1.
2.
3.
4.
5.
6.
7.
8.
9.
10.

Most people think this kind of care is challenging and rewarding but what about the client? Feeling empathy for someone who is critically ill can be difficult when you have never experienced it. Picture yourself as very ill and dependent on others to meet all your needs.

A. What would you want from your nurse if you were a critically ill client who was voiceless?

B. What do you think you would want to say most if you were voiceless?

C. How would you communicate your needs such as pain?

D. If you were voiceless, what is most important to you?

Discussion

Write a brief summary of what you think it might be like to be voiceless. What would you like your nurse to do or say?

2.   Responding to Situations

Below are situations in which you might find yourself as you interact with critically ill clients who are voiceless in the clinical setting. These situations are posed to help you better understand the process of therapeutic interaction.

A.   Your client, Mr. Jackson, is 18 years old and admitted to the Emergency Room after being transported by an emergency vehicle from the scene of an accident. He was a healthy, African American man who recently graduated from high school when he was hit by an automobile while riding his motorcycle. When you conduct an initial assessment, you note that he is unable to speak.

✳ What do you think Mr. Jackson feels in this situation?

✳ What might you feel in this situation?

✳ What would you say and or do that might be helpful for Mr. Jackson?

B.   Mr. Bentley, a 65-year-old White, married man with an 8th-grade education, was transported to the hospital because his wife feared he was having a stroke. While in the emergency room, his condition deteriorated and he was admitted to the critical care unit with a tracheostomy.

✳ What might he be feeling in this situation?

✳ What will you say to him when you first meet?

Discussion

In your self-assessment notebook, summarize what you have learned in doing this exercise. What kinds of feelings do you experience in caring for critically ill clients? How do you handle those feelings? What would you like to change about the way you approach critically ill clients?

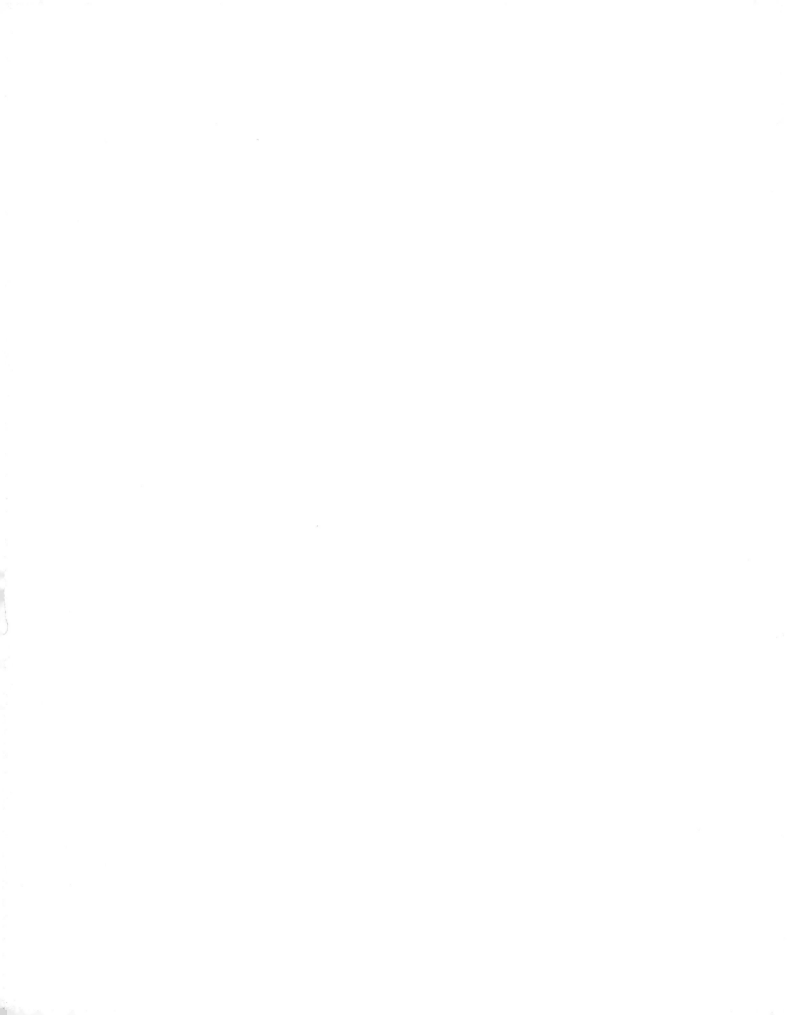

Communicating With Clients With Psychiatric Illnesses

Christine L. Williams, DNSc, RN, BC

OBJECTIVE

1. To discuss the importance of communication as a therapeutic strategy for clients with severe psychiatric illnesses
2. To compare and contrast communication approaches to clients experiencing varying symptoms of severe psychiatric illness
3. To analyze barriers to therapeutic communication with clients who experience psychiatric symptoms

INTRODUCTION

Nurses may care for clients with mental illness in a variety of locations, including inclient psychiatric units, community settings, and urgent care. These clients experience the same medical illnesses, accidents, surgical procedures, and need for primary care as other clients. Individuals may exhibit symptoms of psychiatric illness during childbirth or in settings where their children receive care. Therefore, all nurses should be prepared for interacting with persons with symptoms of mental illness.

There are multiple causes of psychiatric illness, including genetic influences, intrauterine and birth trauma, and environmental factors. Nurses use a variety of strategies to work with this population, including therapeutic milieu, group therapy, one-to-one relationships, and somatic therapies. This chapter focuses on verbal and nonverbal therapeutic techniques the nurse can use when interacting with clients with psychiatric illnesses regardless of setting.

When clients are suffering from mental illness, successful communication can be challenging. Nurses must adapt their approach to the symptoms that clients display. Because the psychiatric client seems so different or so difficult to reach, nurses frequently experience anxiety when they begin working with this population. Caregivers' (both family and professional) emotional reactions to clients with schizophrenia have been studied extensively.[1] Caregiver hostility and lack of warmth have been significantly related to negative client outcomes such as relapse and rehospitalization. Nurses' unrealistic expectations of clients and lack of understanding of symptoms contribute to their negative attitudes and lack of caring.

In his writings about the challenges of understanding the client with schizophrenia, Harry Stack Sullivan[2] reminded readers that clients with psychiatric illness are more similar to us than we realize. He also wrote about the pain of clients' loneliness and isolation, claiming that loneliness is the only emotion that is more painful than anxiety.[2] All clients need relationships, and relationships have the potential to bolster self-worth and increase self-esteem.[3] When nurses focus on what they have in common with their clients, such as the need for love and acceptance, the need for emotional security, and the need for positive relationships with others, they are more likely to be supportive and positive in their approach.

Peplau wrote that the goal of communication is to develop a common understanding between people in order to develop a relationship.[4] In Peplau's view, the relationship between nurse and client was intended to be corrective. For example, when nurses help clients to clarify unclear messages, they help to correct their confused thoughts. Today, nurses focus on creating behavior change in clients.[3] Facilitating health-promoting behaviors in clients with mental illness begins with successful communication and relationship building.

Since many psychiatric illnesses share the same symptoms, this chapter is organized around psychiatric symptoms and the communication strategies appropriate with clients experiencing those symptoms. These strategies are intended to guide nurses to respond in helpful ways to clients who seem very different and are often difficult to understand.

Antipsychotic drugs that alter the biochemistry of the brain can decrease or even eliminate symptoms. Treating psychiatric symptoms with psychoactive drugs is an important component of a comprehensive approach to clients with severe psychiatric illness. Not all clients treated with antipsychotics or other psychiatric drugs will be relieved of their symptoms; therefore, other therapeutic strategies will remain an important component of their long-term care.

CHARACTERISTICS OF MENTAL DISORDERS

According to the 2000 *Diagnostic and Statistical Manual of Mental Disorders*,[5] being psychotic can be defined as experiencing delusions and hallucinations when the person does not understand that these are symptoms and therefore not real. Clients with psychoses and other serious psychiatric conditions are the focus of this chapter.

One of the most common manifestations of psychosis, schizophrenia, has an impressive list of symptoms to become acquainted with before communication is likely to be successful. Lego wrote that schizophrenia presented the greatest challenge to the nurse's ability to communicate.[6] The symptoms associated with schizophrenia are also common in many other mental disorders, although some symptoms will be more dominant in one disorder than others. For example, an individual with Alzheimer's disease may experience similar symptoms to the person with schizophrenia (hallucinations, delusions, and mood symptoms). In Alzheimer's disease, paranoid delusions and visual hallucinations may be dominant, whereas in schizophrenia, auditory hallucinations and grandiose delusions are most prominent. In the following discussion, symptoms will be categorized as negative, positive, cognitive, and mood related.

Creating a feeling of interpersonal safety for the client is the first step in a therapeutic interaction. Many clients with psychiatric illness withdraw from others or are difficult to engage in a relationship. The nurse can begin by acting in ways that are non-threatening. Sitting quietly at a distance of 10 to 12 feet communicates availability. Being available and observant without being obvious creates a presence that is non-demanding. In this atmosphere of acceptance, the client is more likely to approach you and to initiate an interaction.

Symptoms can become habitual for persons experiencing severe psychiatric illness and nurses must demonstrate patience as clients struggle to give up familiar ways of relating.[7] A gentle, supportive approach is most useful for bringing about change. An important principle is repetition. Any one strategy must be used over and over to have beneficial effects. Nurses sometimes wonder if their efforts will have any effect on client communication. Some worry about saying anything in case a poorly worded response might cause harm to the client. No one response is likely to have lasting impact. Consistency and persistence are necessary to gradually bring about positive change.[8]

RELATING TO CLIENTS WITH POSITIVE SYMPTOMS

Positive symptoms are assessment findings that would be absent if clients were healthy. The positive symptoms of psychiatric illness include abnormal findings such as hallucinations and delusions.

Hallucinations

Hallucinations are perceptions that are not based in reality.[5] Hallucinations can be understood as having some meaning beyond the literal description of the hallucinations themselves.[7] As nurses become more familiar with their clients, they may begin to understand more about the psychological issues their clients struggle with by understanding the specific meaning of a hallucination for a specific client.

According to Peplau,[9] hallucinations develop gradually in psychiatric illness, beginning when individuals call to mind thoughts of a comforting image during threatening experiences. When the stressful experience ends, individuals forget the comforting image or voice until the next stressful experience arises and the comforting image or voice is needed again. Gradually, this process becomes habitual and extends to situations in which the individual does not deliberately conjure up the comforting image or voice, but it comes to mind unexpectedly. The individual seems to be losing control. Something that brought relief during times of stress becomes a stressor in itself. As experiences of the image or voice increase and become uncontrollable, individuals distort the experience. Now the image or voice seems to be originating outside the self. Further distortions continue and the comforting image becomes very frightening.

From a neurobiological perspective, brain activity during hallucinations differs from normal. Transferring neural messages between different parts of the brain is thought to be impaired in schizophrenia. For the person who is hallucinating, thoughts that are expressed in words may seem to come from a source outside the person when in fact they are self-generated.[10] In light of this fragmentation in the transfer of information, it is understandable that the client who is hallucinating will insist that the "voices" are not his or her own thoughts. Arguing with the client about the source of the voices will foster the client's distrust. Accepting the client's experience as being "real" for him or her can foster a trusting relationship. As a therapeutic relationship develops, the client can learn more about hallucinations as a symptom of illness.

For persons who develop hallucinations during physical illness (eg, while withdrawing from alcohol or other substances), the hallucinations may be fleeting and much less organized than hallucinatory experiences of clients with schizophrenia. Such hallucinations tend to be visual and are associated with delirium (see Chapter 7 for a discussion of therapeutic communication with clients experiencing delirium).

Hallucinations are common during dementia, such as in the later stages of Alzheimer's disease. The verbal strategies that follow are appropriate for clients with hallucinations arising during delirium and dementia, as well as during psychiatric illness.

In order to begin helping clients to recognize their own thoughts, nurses must avoid reinforcing the hallucination as something that originates outside the person. When asking clients to describe the experience, ask "What is this voice you tell me you hear saying?" rather than "What does the voice say?" It is important to acknowledge clients' experiences, although you do not experience the same thing. For example, "You are telling me you hear a voice and I know this is very real for you, but I do not hear it." With a response such as this, nurses convey acceptance of clients' experiences and contrast those experiences with their own. The goal is to encourage clients to question the reality of the symptom. When the experience is recognized as a symptom rather than external reality, client anxiety decreases.

Delusions

Delusions are false beliefs that may be fleeting but are often stable over time.[5] Clients cannot be persuaded to give up false beliefs despite evidence to the contrary. Arguing with clients serves no useful purpose and may be harmful to the therapeutic relationship. Directly challenging delusions increases clients' anxiety and, thus, increases their need to maintain the delusion. The delusion can be used to help the nurse recognize a client's unmet emotional needs. For example, clients who, in reality, feel worthless may insist they are celebrities or important religious figures (grandiosity). The delusion may be an exaggeration of what clients really feel. For example, clients who feel threatened and unsafe speak of delusions of being watched, stalked, chased, or even poisoned (paranoid delusions).

The nurse conveys acceptance of the person while avoiding confirmation of the delusion. Addressing the underlying feeling helps the client feel more secure rather than challenged.

RELATING TO CLIENTS WITH NEGATIVE SYMPTOMS

The negative symptoms of psychiatric illness require special attention as well. Negative symptoms refer to characteristics of a healthy person that would

Case Example

Mrs. Jackson, age 90, lives in a nursing home and is diagnosed with Alzheimer's disease. She tells the nurse she does not want to come to the dining room for lunch because "they are trying to poison me." The nurse notices that Mrs. Jackson becomes highly anxious when taken from her room to the noisy, crowded dining area. She demonstrates understanding by responding, "You seem very frightened, Mrs. Jackson." She asks the nursing assistant to bring Mrs. Jackson's lunch to her room to see if this might decrease her anxiety.

be expected findings during a mental health assessment. Negative symptoms relate to the absence of healthy responses or behaviors and include flat affect (lack of affect), alogia (lack of speech), and avolition (lack of motivation).

Flat Affect

A lack of nonverbal expressiveness when communicating can make it difficult to understand what the client is feeling. In studies comparing the emotional experiences of individuals diagnosed with schizophrenia to individuals without a psychiatric diagnosis, both groups reported similar emotions when watching film clips. The individuals with schizophrenia did not appear to be reacting emotionally due to flat affect but they reported similar subjective experiences. When interacting with individuals with flat affect, assume that clients experience a range of emotions but are unable to express them nonverbally.[11]

Clients with flat affect lack the facial expressiveness and gestures that normally communicate moment-to-moment changes in emotions.[5] These clients may avoid eye contact as well. Since nurses rely on nonverbal communication to convey emotions, other means will be necessary to discover what the client is feeling. Listening for themes in conversation and asking for validation are helpful in identifying client concerns and emotions. Notice words that express emotions, such as "upset," "frustrated," "excited," and so on. Ask the client to elaborate.

Alogia

Alogia or poverty of speech is another negative symptom.[5] Alogia includes speech in which few words are used and few ideas are expressed. Alogia

can progress to mutism or complete lack of verbal expression. These symptoms can be aggravated by side effects of medication or depression. The result is a client who is unable or unwilling to communicate verbally.[12] Clients who do not communicate verbally or who use very little speech may be easily ignored. Understanding their needs requires effort and patience.

When clients are silent, too often nurses rush to fill the silence with a question. Clients can be encouraged to formulate their own thoughts by allowing them time to reflect in silence. Avoid interrupting clients' silence when you believe they are thinking and eventually they may respond independently. Informing clients that you will spend a specific brief amount of time with them (whether they are verbal or not) sets the stage for a trusting relationship. When trust develops, clients who were nonverbal may begin to interact.

Questioning can influence the amount of spontaneous communication clients use. If nurses ask closed-ended questions (questions that can be answered with "yes" or "no" or one word), they unknowingly discourage elaboration. When clients provide a one-word answer, nurses must think of other strategies to encourage verbalization. Open-ended questions that request specific information, such as "who?" "what?" "where?" and "when?" are more helpful. These questions foster descriptions of client experiences that can be used to examine patterns of behavior that are problematic for clients.

Avoid the use of questions that begin with "how?" or "why?" since these questions are so difficult to answer that a helpful response is unlikely. Clients may give an answer, but if the response is carefully examined, it is usually not directly related to the question. "How?" and "why?" questions require a degree of sophisticated reflection and analysis of experiences that clients with psychiatric illness cannot usually provide.

Avolition

Avolition is another negative symptom that includes lack of motivation and apathy.[5] Clients with psychiatric illnesses may seem unmotivated to participate in care or even to dress and bathe themselves when abnormalities in neuromotor function may contribute to their lack of action.[11] Nurses need to recognize their own emotional responses to clients who seem unmotivated to care for themselves. Frustration and anger are common responses to these symptoms and must be recognized and discussed with another nurse or supervisor. When feelings of irritation go unrecognized, the nurse may unknowingly convey lack of acceptance to the client. It may be helpful to remember that these behaviors are symptoms, and when clients improve, they do participate in their care.

Avoid confronting the client who is apathetic but use gentle encouragement. Remember that this lack of energy is discouraging for the client as well. Provide opportunities for the client to get involved in a nonthreatening manner such as playing a game of dominoes with other clients and inviting the client to participate. Often clients refuse participation at first but when the nurse is accepting and conveys warmth, clients may decide to participate at a later time. Providing opportunities for small successes can build a client's confidence to try more challenging activities.

RELATING TO CLIENTS WITH COGNITIVE IMPAIRMENT

Cognitive impairment that is observed in clients with psychiatric illness is reflected in disorganized speech, vague language, and automatic knowing. Nurses must adapt their communication to clients' impaired thinking.[4]

Disorganized Speech

Cognitive dysfunction may be very evident in the impaired language of the client with psychiatric symptoms. Impairments are more evident when the client is faced with a challenge or becomes anxious.[12] In discussions of threatening topics, clients may seem to avoid direct communication.[8] Avoidance can become a habitual way of interacting. Clients may tell nurses "I can't remember," "I don't know," or "I can't think" when they are discussing anxiety-provoking situations. To help clients communicate their experiences effectively, suggest that clients tell you about specific situations. For example, the nurse states, "Tell me what happened just before you came to the hospital this morning."

Nurses can effectively influence *continuity of thought* by asking questions selectively that maintain the client's focus of attention on a theme or topic.[9] Changing topics reinforces scattered thought. For example, the client begins to discuss a conflict between herself and another client. The nurse responds by asking how well she slept last night.

Vague Language

Vague language such as the use of pronouns must be clarified by the nurse in order to increase clear communication and mutual understanding. For example, the client states, "They are after me!" The therapeutic response is to question who the client is referring to: "Who are they?" or "Who do you mean?" Each time the client uses an unclear pronoun, the nurse should ask for clarification. The nurse may need to ask many times before getting a specific response, such as the name of a person. The goal is to have the client identify specifically who is referred to in order to clarify vague thoughts. When nurses fail to question the use of unclear messages, they reinforce this communication pattern.

Automatic Knowing

Automatic knowing is another thought pattern that is characteristic of clients with psychiatric illness.[3] This pattern involves the belief that others know what you think without any explanation. It is communicated in statements such as "You know?" or "You know what I mean?" When clients assume that others know their thoughts, it is unhelpful because it interferes with communication. If clients continue to believe another can "know" without being told, there is no need to communicate verbally, and these beliefs may extend to other ways that another can influence their thoughts. Clarification by the nurse is necessary each time the client implies that the nurse automatically knows. The nurse may respond, "No, I don't know. Tell me."[8] It is important to use a supportive tone of voice and facial expressions conveying warmth and acceptance.

RELATING TO CLIENTS WITH MOOD SYMPTOMS

Negative moods (dysphoria) are also associated with schizophrenia and many other mental disorders. Anhedonia (lack of interest or lack of pleasure), negative self-views, and anger are all common symptoms that the nurse will encounter.[5]

Dysphoria

Clients with dysphoria often project an overall feeling of sadness or depression. The client may be able to smile on occasion or appreciate a joke, but they are depressed most of the time, day after day. The nurse may be uncomfortable with this mood and try to bring about a change with a cheerful approach. This approach is usually ineffective and the client may smile because it is expected rather than because he or she is genuinely more cheerful. When the nurse matches the intensity of his or her emotions to the client's, he or she is perceived as more understanding. For example, if the client is quiet and sad when approached by the nurse, the nurse can mirror this with a subdued demeanor. Offering to be available as a quiet presence or for quiet conversation is more effective than burdening the client with excessive talk. Silence can be used effectively to encourage the client to respond at his or her own pace.

Anhedonia

The inability to experience pleasure or even complete lack of interest in activities that one used to enjoy is anhedonia. The *negativity* displayed when the client has anhedonia can evoke strong reactions in nurses. As in avolition, nurses must examine their own feelings to be sure that their responses convey acceptance of the client as a person despite his or her behavior. Nurses must avoid personalizing when clients seem to reject their efforts to help and remember that the client's cognitive dysfunction contributes to lack of expressiveness.

Clients who are negative refuse to participate in pleasurable activities, such as taking a walk, conversations with others despite loneliness and isolation, and even activities of daily living. In order to respond constructively, nurses must avoid giving alternatives that will lead to unacceptable choices. For example, "Would you like to get out of bed?" places the nurse in a difficult position when the client answers, "No." Instead, use a direct approach: "It's time to get up now." The client can still refuse but is less likely to do so. Another example is the nurse who asks, "Would you like to talk now?" A better approach would be to state, "Tell me about yourself." This directness is more likely to be rewarded with an answer, particularly if the nurse waits silently until the client answers.

Case Example

A young mother describes an experience in which she was unable to console her newborn. Kara, age 24, states that she is determined to be a better mother than her own mother was. This is her first child and she tells the nurse that she wants to do "everything right". Each time the infant cries, Kara picks her up and tries to comfort her. When she is unsuccessful, Kara confides that she feels "like a failure". Her "all or nothing" thinking about motherhood is contributing to her feelings of sadness and defeat. Kara believes that the infant should never cry or at least that a mother should always be able to determine why her baby is crying and to soothe her infant. Kara's attitude changed when the nurse provided information about infant crying. She came to understand that she could not remove every discomfort for her infant and that different cries had different meanings. With this information, she focused on learning more about her infant's cries and trying to discriminate among them. In her encounter with the nurse, she was assisted to examine her negative self-views and question her own conclusions. As a result, her self-view improved.

Negative Self-Views

Dysphoria is accompanied by negative self-views. When the client states, "I'm no good," the nurse may rush to dispute this negative self-evaluation by saying, "That's not true. I think you are a wonderful person." This response is unlikely to have any positive effect. The self is very resistant to change and is designed to reject evaluations that are incompatible with previously held views.[7] Instead, clients must be guided in evaluating their conclusions and the methods they used to arrive at those conclusions. The process involves having clients describe one experience at a time in which they concluded something negative about themselves. As individual experiences are examined objectively, the overall negative conclusion is questioned by the client.

Anger

Irritability, hostility, and anger commonly accompany mood symptoms and can interfere with nurses' attempts to develop therapeutic relationships. When nurses approach hostile clients, they may be more concerned about their own emotional well-being and personal safety than about clients' needs. Nurses must focus on anger as a symptom rather than a personal attack. A calm, matter-of-fact approach is needed to communicate that the nurse accepts the client as a person. Nurses need to communicate that they will not avoid or isolate angry clients but will continue to work with them to understand their concerns.

CONCLUSION

Persons with mental illness are often isolated by stigma. Lack of social contacts and loneliness account for much of their poor quality of life. Their inability to function in social roles such as work, parenting, and even leisure activities creates a critical need for therapeutic relationship building.[13] Nurses with the communication skills to reach out to clients with mental illness can play a critical role in improving clients' quality of life.

REFERENCES

1. Willetts LE, Leff J. Expressed emotion and schizophrenia: the efficacy of a staff training programme. *Journal of Advanced Nursing.* 1997;26:1125-1133.
2. Sullivan HS. *The Interpersonal Theory of Psychiatry.* New York: WW Norton & Co; 1954.
3. Peplau HE. Peplau's theory of interpersonal relations. *Nursing Science Quarterly.* 1997;10(4):162-167.
4. Peplau HE. *Interpersonal Relations in Nursing.* New York: Putnam; 1952.
5. American Psychiatric Association. *Diagnostic and Statistical Manual of Mental Disorders, Test Revision.* 4th ed. Washington, DC: American Psychiatric Association; 2000.
6. Lego S. The one-to-one nurse-patient relationship. *Archives of Psychiatric Nursing.* 1999;35(4):4-18.
7. Reynolds WJ. Peplau's theory in practice. *Nursing Science Quarterly.* 1997;10(4):168-170.
8. Gregg DE. Hildegard E. Peplau: her contributions. *Perspectives in Psychiatric Care.* 1997;35(3):10-19.
9. Peplau HE. *Basic Principles of Patient Counseling.* Philadelphia: Smith Kline & French Laboratories; 1964.
10. Stern E, Silbersweig DA. Neural mechanisms underlying hallucinations in schizophrenia: the role of abnormal frontal-temporal interactions. In: Lenzenweger MF, Dworkin RH, eds. *Origins and Development of Schizophrenia.* Washington, DC: American Psychological Association; 1998.
11. Dworkin RH, Oster H, Clark SC, White SR. Affective expression and affective experience in schizophrenia. In: Lenzenweger MF, Dworkin RH, eds. *Origins and Development of Schizophrenia.* Washington, DC: American Psychological Association; 1998.
12. Walker EF, Baum KM, Diforio D. Developmental changes in the behavioral expression of vulnerability for schizophrenia. In: Lenzenweger MF, Dworkin RH, eds. *Origins and Development of Schizophrenia.* Washington, DC: American Psychological Association; 1998.
13. McDonald J, Badger TA. Social function in persons with schizophrenia. *Journal of Psychosocial Nursing and Mental Health Services.* 2002;40(6):42-50.

EXERCISES

1. Self-Assessment

Caring for clients with severe and persistent mental disorders can be anxiety-provoking. Much of what students expect about clients with psychiatric disorders is based on myths or lay knowledge. Use the following exercises to help explore your beliefs about mental illness.

* Have you ever been diagnosed with a psychiatric disorder?

* If so, do you let others know that you have had these experiences?

* If not, is there anyone you know personally who is diagnosed with mental illness?

* What do you think is the cause your (his or her) problem?

* What do you think can be done (if anything) to help him or her (or you)?

* When did you first learn about mental illness?

* What did you learn from your family about mental illness?

* What did you learn in elementary or high school about mental illness?

Discussion

In your self-assessment notebook, summarize what you have learned in doing this exercise. How do your earlier ideas about mental illness differ from your understanding today? How have your earlier experiences influenced your choices about working with this population?

2. Responding to Situations

A. You are a nurse in labor and delivery. A woman with a diagnosis of bipolar disorder is being admitted in active labor. The nurse manager assigns you to care for her.

* What might your feelings be in this situation?

* What are your expectations about how this client will manage in labor?

B. You are a home health nurse who is assigned to visit Mr. Rogers, who is diagnosed with schizophrenia. He is a 57-year-old Vietnam veteran living in an assisted living facility. Mr. Rogers has a history of frequent rehospitalization after refusing his antipsychotic medication.

* Is there really anything you can do that will make a difference in health outcomes for Mr. Rogers?

* What challenges do you expect in establishing a relationship with this client?

* What rewards might there be in caring for Mr. Rogers?

Discussion

In your self-assessment notebook, summarize what you think about caring for clients with severe and persistent mental illness. What feelings can you identify that might influence your approach to such clients?

3. Practice Exercises

Write the therapeutic response to the client statements below.

Client Statement	Your Therapeutic Response
"I'm no prisoner, I am St. Jude. They are following me."	
"It's criminal! I won't wait till you shoot me, I'll shoot first."	
"It's no use, I never do anything right."	
"The voices are telling me I'm the chosen one."	
"You know when the doctor will discharge me, why don't you tell me?"	

Index